Psychotherapeutic Interventions for Adults with Brain Injury or Stroke

Psychotherapeutic Interventions for Adults with Brain Injury or Stroke: A Clinician's Treatment Resource

Edited by

Karen G. Langer, Ph.D.,
Linda Laatsch, Ph.D., &
Lisa Lewis, Ph.D.

Psychosocial Press
Madison, Connecticut

Library of Congress Cataloging-in-Publication Data

Psychotherapeutic interventions for adults with brain injury or stroke
: a clinician's treatment resource / edited by Karen G. Langer, Linda
Laatsch & Lisa Lewis.
    p.   cm.
  Includes bibliographical references and indexes.
  ISBN 1-887841-23-7
  1. Brain—Wounds and injuries—Treatment.   2. Cerebrovascular
disease—Patients—Rehabilitation.   3. Psychotherapy.   I. Langer,
Karen G.   II. Laatsch, Linda.
  [DNLM: 1. Psychotherapy—methods.   2. Brain Injuries—psychology.
3. Cerebrovascular Disorders—psychology.   4. Depression—therapy.
5. Transference (Psychology).   WM 420 P97424 1999]
RC387.5.P77   1999
616.89'14—dc21
DNLM/DLC
for Library of Congress   99-24556
                                                              CIP

Manufactured in the United States of America

Table of Contents

Contributors

Robert W. Butler, Ph.D., ABPP, is Associate Professor, Department of Pediatrics, Oregon Health Sciences University; Director, Pediatric Neuropsychology Clinic, Child Development and Rehabilitation Center, Oregon Health Sciences University, Portland, Oregon.

Leonard Diller, Ph.D., ABPP, is Director, Psychology and Behavioral Sciences, Rusk Institute of Rehabilitation Medicine, New York University Medical Center, Professor of Rehabilitation Medicine, New York University School of Medicine, New York City.

Robert M. Gordon, Psy.D., is Director, Intern Training, Rusk Institute of Rehabilitation Medicine, New York University Medical Center; Clinical Assistant Professor of Rehabilitation Medicine, New York University School of Medicine, New York City.

Bennett Hanig, Ph.D., is a Consultant, RHR International, New York City.

Allen W. Heinemann, Ph.D., is a Professor, Department of Physical Medicine and Rehabilitation, Northwestern University Medical School; Director of Rehabilitation Services Evaluation Unit, Rehabilitation Institute, Chicago; Associate Director of Research, Rehabilitation Institute, Chicago.

Linda Laatsch, Ph.D., is Associate Professor of Psychology, Department of Rehabilitation Medicine and Restorative Medical Sciences, University of Illinois College of Medicine, Chicago.

Donna M. Langenbahn, Ph.D., is Supervisor, Adult Outpatient Neuropsychology Service, Rusk Institute of Rehabilitation

Medicine, New York University Medical Center; Clinical Assistant Professor of Rehabilitation Medicine, New York University School of Medicine, New York City.

Karen G. Langer, Ph.D., ABMP, is Supervisor of Psychology, Inpatient Services, Rusk Institute of Rehabilitation Medicine, New York University Medical Center; Clinical Assistant Professor of Rehabilitation Medicine, New York University School of Medicine, New York City.

Lisa Lewis, Ph.D., is Director of Psychology and Director of Neuropsychological Services, Menninger Foundation, Topeka, Kansas.

Laurence Miller, Ph.D., is a licensed psychologist and brain/behavior consultant, specializing in clinical and forensic neuropsychology, psychotherapy and rehabilitation, crisis intervention and trauma therapy, and workplace relations and management training.

Frank J. Padrone, Ph.D., is Assistant Director of Psychology, Director, Inpatient Services, Rusk Institute of Rehabilitation Medicine, New York University Medical Center; Clinical Associate Professor of Rehabilitation Medicine, New York University School of Medicine, New York City.

Mary Sano, Ph.D., is a consultant, Physical Medicine Associates, Jacksonville, Florida; Associate Professor of Clinical Neuropsychology, Columbia University, College of Physicians and Surgeons, New York City.

Paul Satz, Ph.D., ABPP, is Professor of Medical Psychology, Department of Psychiatry and Biobehavioral Sciences, UCLA Medical School; Director, Neuropsychology Program, Neuropsychiatric Institute, UCLA Medical School.

Mary F. Schmidt, Ph.D., is a Clinical Neuropsychologist, Rehabilitation Center, Lutheran General Hospital, Park Ridge, Illinois; Senior Clinical Research Associate, Rehabilitation Institute of Chicago.

Rose Lynn Sherr, Ph.D., ABPP, is Director, Outpatient Psychology, Rusk Institute of Rehabilitation Medicine, New York University Medical Center; Clinical Associate Professor of Rehabilitation Medicine, New York University School of Medicine, New York City.

Dvorah Simon, Ph.D., is Senior Psychologist, Adult Outpatient Neuropsychology Service, Rusk Institute of Rehabilitation Medicine, New York University Medical Center; Clinical Assistant Professor of Rehabilitation Medicine, New York University School of Medicine, New York City.

Robert W. Sury, M.D., is a partner in Physical Medicine Associates, Jacksonville, Florida.

Joseph Weinberg, Ph.D., is Staff Psychologist, Rusk Institute of Rehabilitation Medicine, New York University Medical Center; Clinical Assistant Professor of Rehabilitation Medicine, New York University School of Medicine, New York City.

Introduction

It is often helpful to view developments in a field within a historical perspective. Until the mid-1980s, little had been written about conducting psychological treatment with patients having traumatic brain injury (TBI), stroke, or other types of acquired brain dysfunction, and much of what had been written suggested that these patients' cognitive deficits would prevent them from taking a full part in the psychotherapeutic process. "Organic Brain Dysfunction" was found on most lists of exclusionary criteria for various forms of individual and group psychotherapy. This attitude of therapeutic nihilism was challenged in 1973 by Leonard Small in his book *Neuropsychodiagnosis in Psychotherapy,* and was soon followed by an increasing number of articles and books constructively addressing the psychological treatment needs of patients with brain injury or stroke (e.g., Ball, 1988; Cicerone, 1989; Langer, 1992; Lewis, 1986; Miller, 1991; Prigatano et al., 1986). It is now commonly recognized that attending to the patient's psychological recovery and growth is as predictive of overall outcome as the rehabilitation of cognitive and physical deficits. It is in the spirit of this recognition that this book is written.

This volume is intended as a practical resource for clinicians who treat brain injury and stroke patients whether in an individual, family, or group psychotherapy format. Our goal is to address the issues that face clinicians who work with these patients. The challenge to the psychotherapist is to adapt traditional approaches to the specific needs of patients with brain injury. These needs are based on the neuropsychological deficits of the patient, as they disrupt linear learning, as well as on the emotional effects that the brain injury has posed. These emotional effects may include primary (i.e., direct) disruptions (e.g., of personality or of affective control, etc., secondary to the brain injury), or secondary effects (i.e., due to the losses incurred by the brain injury and the subsequent need to adapt to altered life circumstances, often in an abrupt and sometimes wrenchingly painful way). These secondary emotional effects may be very substantial and significant in their impact on the person, in terms of former and current identity, sense of competence and mastery, and in short, on all of what makes up one's sense of self. All of these may be challenged by the brain injury, sometimes altered in a fundamental way, and sometimes merely reconsidered. The reconsideration itself, an integral part of the psychotherapeutic process, can also be the foundation for mature review of personal assumptions, beliefs, and values, and hence for personal growth.

We have concentrated entirely on acquired brain impairment, as opposed to congenital dysfunction, since the two pose very different issues for patient and family. For purposes of clarity, we restrict our discussion to the brain injury and stroke patient populations, though we acknowledge that many of the principles described will also be applicable to patients with neoplastic or infectious diseases of the central nervous system, or patients with organic brain syndromes secondary to substance abuse or toxic exposure, and, to a lesser degree, patients with primary degenerative dementias.

The reader will be able both to explore the challenges of psychotherapy with the patient with stroke or brain injury in general, and focus on recent developments in treatment applications and clinical approaches. The topics covered in this volume are by no means exhaustive of the array of diagnostic and treatment considerations, but they are broad based and reflect diversity in approach.

We have divided the book into sections based on conceptual groupings. The first section includes the background, history, and ethical issues involved in treating the patient with brain injury or stroke. Key orienting and overview chapters are written by Drs. Robert Sury and Mary Sano who provide an accessible and clinically focused account of the range of deficits and syndromes resulting from damage to the dominant and nondominant cerebral hemispheres. Dr. Laurence Miller then cogently describes the development of psychotherapeutic approaches to the patient with brain injury/stroke, and Dr. Robert Gordon discusses the crucial issues of what can be accomplished in treatment to help the patient in both ethical and practical terms.

The next section deals with implications of emotional reactions, defensive functions, and countertransferential issues in therapeutic treatment of these patients. The first two chapters focus on the clinical phenomena which pose the biggest challenge in the treatment of the patient with brain injury/stroke and can, when successfully addressed, make the difference between poor and favorable treatment outcomes: depression and unawareness of deficit. Dr. Karen Langer addresses the multifaceted problem of unawareness of deficit and the treatment approaches that can lead patient and therapist to be mutually allied in a shared understanding of the problems, their causes, and their solutions. Drs. Robert Butler and Paul Satz provide an excellent guide to navigating differential diagnostic dilemmas and employing effective treatment strategies when working with the patient manifesting depressive mood and affect. Dr. Lisa Lewis, coming from a psychoanalytic perspective, describes the common transference and countertransference paradigms that emerge in therapy with the patient with brain injury/stroke and how they can be put to therapeutic gain rather than leading to derailment of the therapeutic enterprise.

A rapprochement between cognitive rehabilitation and traditional psychotherapy is undertaken in the next set of chapters. Dr. Linda Laatsch addresses, in clinically relevant terms, how cognitive retraining and psychotherapy can be blended with synergistic effects on patient experience and treatment outcome. Drs. Joseph Weinberg and Leonard Diller, two pioneers in the field of rehabilitation, discuss and illustrate their state-of-the-art clinical approach to treating patients with unilateral visual neglect, an approach which incorporates psychotherapeutic approaches to resistance and defense into an integrated rehabilitative effort.

The final section of the book is devoted to treatment approaches that are designed to meet unique or specialized patient needs, or those of the family. Drs. Donna Langenbahn, Rose Lynn Sherr, Dvorah Simon, and Bennett Hanig astutely describe the power of group psychotherapy in which the patient with brain injury/stroke can be lifted from painful isolation by a growing sense of deeply shared common experience with other group members, and how this can serve as the catalyst for broader social and interpersonal reintegration. Dr. Frank Padrone discusses how family dynamics can be destabilized by the shattering impact of brain injury/stroke and how a restoration of meaning and cohesiveness can occur in a family therapy process. Drs. Mary Schmidt and Allen Heinemann address a topic which has too long been neglected given that it plays such a powerfully undermining role in recovery and treatment outcome: substance abuse. Practical assessment tools, means of establishing a multidisciplinary treatment program in the reader's home community, and up-to-date psychotherapeutic approaches are offered which address the unique needs of the patient with brain injury/stroke who abuses alcohol and other drugs.

It is hoped then that the reader will find this a rich and useful text for reviewing the history and current considerations in psychotherapy with the patient with brain injury/stroke and in the diagnostic and conceptual challenges that pertain to their treatment. It is the aim of the authors to collect and expand our knowledge in this growing and important field of practice.

Psychotherapy, at its essence, is about the creation and discovery of meaning. For the patient with any form of brain injury, the principles described in the following chapters will allow for the discovery of meaning which can recreate a sense of continuity to their lives, linking past (insight into the brain injury/stroke), present (insight into current deficits, interpersonal patterns, and adaptive capacities), and future (through creation of realistic hope and increased self-efficacy which foster goal attainment). As coeditors of this book, we would like to express our appreciation to our patients, who have been the driving force and inspiration behind this book, to our colleagues whose insights have been powerfully educative, and to our families and friends, who have been a constant source of support, wisdom and encouragement.

K. G. Langer, L. L. Laatsch, and L. Lewis, Editors

REFERENCES

Ball, J. D. (1988). Psychotherapy with head-injured patients. *Journal of Medical Psychotherapy, 1,* 15–22.

Cicerone, K. D. (1989). Psychotherapeutic intervention with traumatically brain-injured patients. *Rehabilitation Psychology, 34,* 105–114.

Langer, K. G. (1992). Psychotherapy with the neuropsychologically impaired adult. *American Journal of Psychotherapy, 46,* 620–639.

Lewis, L. (1986). Individual psychotherapy with patients having combined psychological and neurological disorders. *Bulletin of the Menninger Clinic, 50,* 75–87.

Miller, L. (1991). Psychotherapy of the brain-injured patient: Principles and practices. *Cognitive Rehabilitation, 9,* 24–30.

Prigatano, G. P., Fordyce, D. J., Zeiner, H. K., Roueche, J. R., Pepping, M., & Wood, B. C. (1986). *Neuropsychological rehabilitation after brain injury.* Baltimore: Johns Hopkins University Press.

Small, L. (1973). *Neuropsychodiagnosis in psychotherapy.* New York: Brunner/Mazel.

PART I

Background, History, and Ethical Considerations

1.

Neuropsychological Impairment: Challenges for Therapeutic Intervention

Robert W. Sury, M.D. and Mary Sano, Ph.D.

Many patients in the rehabilitation setting have neurologic injuries that result in both behavioral and physical impairments. Neuropsychological deficits, affective disturbances, and behavioral problems can occur. To a great degree the pattern of deficit is determined by the location of the injury. The organization of the brain and the spinal cord is such that specific injuries predict relatively specific patterns of deficit. The physical challenges that are commonly associated with neuropsychological impairment result from the paresis, plegia, and cranial nerve injuries that can occur with serious brain injury. Physical challenges for the patient with spinal cord injury, which include paralysis and hemiplegia, are often accompanied by neuropsychological deficits which may result from minor head injury (Davidoff, Roth, & Richards, 1992). These injuries may initially go undetected because of the presence of severe physical disability. Recent work had suggested that neuropsychological impairment from mild head injury is common and can increase the challenge that the patient faces in dealing with his physical limitations.

3

Neuropsychological impairment is also a common sequela of stroke, and the accompanying challenges must often be considered in the context of advanced age. The organization of the brain determines the deficit, and therefore common patterns are seen regardless of the etiology of the deficit. This chapter will discuss common patterns of neuropsychological deficits and physical impairment which can be seen in the rehabilitation setting. This work is not meant as a comprehensive review of the consequences of neurologic injury. Rather, it represents a selection of commonly observed patterns of deficits which represent a challenge to psychotherapeutic interventions.

ORGANIZATION OF THE BRAIN AND SPINAL CORD

The brain may be divided into two hemispheres. The dominant hemisphere refers to the half which controls language. In right-handed individuals, this is the left hemisphere. The left hemisphere is also the dominant one for 60% of left-handed individuals. Motor control and sensation of one side of the body are controlled by the opposite half of the brain. This contralateral representation of motor control and sensation holds true for the upper and lower extremities and for some facial muscles. Other facial and upper body muscles are controlled by the cranial nerves which have ipsilateral (same side) representation in the brain. In addition to motor control, sensation, and language, other cognitive and behavioral functions have also been associated with specific brain locations.

The brain is further divided into lobes which have associated cognitive and physical functions. Motor control and sensation for the entire body are represented on the cortical surface of the brain in a highly organized fashion. The motor strip refers to an area on the precentral gyrus of the frontal lobes, which extends from the midline between the two hemispheres and along the outside of each hemisphere. The sensory cortex refers to the area along the postcentral gyrus of the parietal lobes and is adjacent and posterior to the motor strip. Representations of motor control and sensation of a given area are adjacent to each other. The lower extremities are represented in the midline between the cerebral hemispheres. Representation of the upper extremities and head is lateral along the surface of the frontal and parietal lobes. The amount of cortical surface associated with a given body part is proportional to the complexity of movement and sensation of that body part. For example, there is a greater surface area on the motor cortex representing the thumb than representing the leg or foot. Damage to the these sites can result in sensory loss or motor weakness.

The frontal lobes have been implicated in executive functions such as planning and initiation as well as inhibitory processes, which negate impulsive expression. Through this mechanism the frontal lobes play an important role in emotional expression.

The temporal lobes are associated with memory abilities with relative specialization for the verbal memory in the left temporal lobe. The dominant temporal lobe is the center of receptive language. Heschl's gyrus, on the superior surface of the left (dominant) temporal lobe, is the primary auditory input for language. There is cortical representation for attributing meaning, source, and location of sounds. The ability to make these associations is critical to the ability to comprehend speech. The right temporal lobe is associated with learning of visually presented material. Time perception has been associated with either temporal lobe.

The parietal lobes are associated with visuospatial abilities and awareness, including awareness of self. Recall that the sensory strip resides in the parietal lobe and is the source of information which allows one to know one's physical position in space. Through frontal connections, this lobe is an integrator of sensory input and meaning. The parietal lobe also plays a role in visual attention, and damage to this area is associated with neglect of or inattention to the contralateral visual field or to one's space.

The occipital lobes are the location of the primary visual cortex. This means that the occipital lobes are ultimately responsible for sight. The representation of visual field is in the contralateral side of the brain. For example, the left visual field, which is captured by the right half of each eye, projects to the right side of the occipital lobe of the brain. The upper portion of the visual field is captured by the lower portion of the eye and projects to the lower portion of the occipital lobe. The lower visual field is captured by the upper portion of each eye and projects to the upper portion of the occipital lobe. Lesions in these areas are associated with loss of primary vision. However, cortical blindness can occur in the absence of awareness of vision loss.

Spinal cord injuries are a common source of physical disability in patients in the rehabilitation setting. The spinal cord is the pathway for all ascending and descending neural connections. The ascending pathways relay sensory input from the periphery to the brain while the descending pathways relay motor instructions from the brain to the peripheral nervous system. The spinal cord gives rise to 31 pairs of spinal nerves: 8 cervical, 12 thoracic, 5 lumbar, 5 sacral, and 1 coccygeal. The spinal cord is not of a single width; there are 2 enlargements. The cervical enlargement carries innervation to and from the upper extremities. The thoracic nerves innervate the intercostal muscles which expand the rib cage to assist in breathing. The lumbar enlargement carries innervation to and from the lower extremities, as well as the bladder, prostate, seminal vesicles, uterus, and external genitalia. Each spinal nerve of the pair is directed to one side of the body with the ventral portion of the nerve containing the descending fibers and the dorsal containing the ascending ones.

Spinal cord injuries can be described as complete or incomplete (Frankel, 1969). In a complete injury, there is total loss of motor control and sensation below the level of the lesion. Several types of incomplete lesions have been described. In sensory-only injuries, there is some sensation present below the level of the lesion but there is complete motor paralysis below that level. Motor-useless injuries are characterized by the presence of some motor power below the level of the lesion, but it is of no practical use to the patient. In motor-useful injuries there is useful motor power below the level of the lesion.

CONDITIONS ASSOCIATED WITH DAMAGE TO THE DOMINANT HEMISPHERE

Aphasia is a common disturbance of dominant hemisphere injury. Aphasia may be divided into expressive versus receptive, which implies that language is both the production and the comprehension of speech. However, while one type may be prominent, individuals often have deficits in both. Expressive aphasia may be described as nonfluent. It is characterized by sparse output, requiring significant effort usually with observed frustration, poor articulation, and disturbed prosody (i.e., abnormal rhythm, inflection, timbre, and melody). Expressive aphasia is usually associated with anterior brain lesions. Milder forms of expressive aphasia may also occur. For example, anomia (word-finding difficulty) may occur without other expressive problems.

Broca's aphasia, an expressive aphasic syndrome, is characterized by nonfluent speech with relatively intact comprehension and poor naming (which may be aided by contextual cuing). Broca's aphasia is usually associated with other physical symptoms resulting from neurological damage in the dominant hemisphere. These patients often have right hemiplegia, sensory loss, or visual field disturbance.

Receptive aphasia may be accompanied by "fluent" speech. In this condition there is often sufficient, even an overabundance of, word production, without articulation deficit and intact prosody, but with an absence of meaning and the presence of significant paraphasic errors (substitution of phonemes or words). This type of disturbance is associated with more posterior damage, usually in the temporal lobe of the dominant hemisphere. Wernicke's aphasia is a receptive aphasia with fluent speech interspersed with paraphasic errors and neologisms. The cardinal features of this aphasia are loss of comprehension and disturbances in repetition. With this aphasia there may be a greater loss of comprehension of spoken or written language. This condition may be accompanied by a superior quadrantopsia, although this may go undetected because of the language impairment. In general, these patients have minimal neurologic findings and their presentation has been mislabeled psychotic.

Unlike Wernicke's aphasia, conduction aphasia is characterized by intact comprehension with a disruption of repetition and fluent, paraphasic speech. Conduction aphasia is thought to result from a disruption of the connections between frontal expressive areas and more posterior receptive areas. This syndrome is often accompanied by ideomotor apraxias of buccofacial and limb motions.

Aphasia can occur with damage to the supplementary motor areas. Such lesions may produce an aphasia which is initially characterized by mutism that resolves to slow, hypophonic, nonfluent speech with echolalia. This condition may be accompanied by weakness and/or sensory loss in the right lower extremity and shoulder, but no deficit in the arm and face. Damage in the adjacent extrasylvian sensory areas has been associated with a fluent aphasia with jargon, echolalia, and poor comprehension. The ability to repeat, coupled with fluent, nonsensical speech, can lead these individuals to be mislabeled schizophrenic.

Other language-based conditions including alexia and agraphia are affected by dominant hemisphere lesions. Neglect refers to the failure to respond to stimuli presented on one side of the body. Right neglect associated with left hemisphere lesions can lead to disturbance in a very basic level of visual processing which gives meaning to the letters. This is important to consider, because the inconsistency between visual abilities and reading abilities may lead to the false interpretations that the reading deficit is functional and not related to the injury.

Agraphia refers to the inability to write, which is not attributable to a pure motor deficit. Agraphia with alexia, in the absence of aphasia, is usually attributable to a left parietal lobe lesion. Lesions of the right parietal lobe lead to a spatial agraphia, which is characterized by duplicate stroke, writing on the right side of the page, and insertion of blank spaces between phonemes (Benson, 1979; Hecaen & Albert, 1978).

Agnosias are disturbances in body schema or body image. They include the loss of recognition or perception of aspects of self. Simultanagnosia refers to the inability to recognize the whole, even though the parts may be well recognized. Lesions in the left occipitotemporal junction have been associated with disturbances. These patients may negotiate their environment without difficulty. However, when presented with a series of stimuli, they may identify some but not all of the stimuli, unless specifically directed to.

CONDITIONS ASSOCIATED WITH DAMAGE TO THE NONDOMINANT HEMISPHERE

In general, visuospatial abilities are attributed to the nondominant (usually right) hemisphere. Neglect may be observed in space or in the person and can occur in many modalities. The neglected side is contralateral to the lesion, but often patients with unilateral neglect will demonstrate subtle deficits on the opposite side. Neglect may occur with damage to either hemisphere. There are several conditions which are unique and prominent with right-brain injuries. Right parietal lobe lesions which may result in left neglect and inattention can sometimes be associated with alexia. This visual deficit interferes with visual processing of the written word. When patients with neglect are asked to read words presented vertically, neglect is not seen (Behrmann, Moskovitch, Black, & Mozer, 1990). However, all patients who make neglect errors also produce orthographically related errors in both the neglected and nonneglected direction, suggesting that the alexia is not merely a deficit in attention, but also involves visual processing. However, the alexia may be seen even when there is no demonstrable visual field defect or visual neglect (Kinsbourne & Warrington, 1962). It may be that reading disturbances reflect complex processing that is sensitive to subtle visuospatial neglect which is not detectable by routine clinical examination. Alexia can be highly disabling, and may occur with few other disturbances. This can challenge the uninformed observer's ability to appreciate the full extent of the deficit.

Deficits in color perception are common with right hemisphere lesions, particularly when a field cut is present. Apperception of color can occur with left hemisphere lesions, particularly when aphasia is present (De Renzi & Spinnler, 1967).

Deficits in the ability to locate an object in space have been associated with lesions of both the left and right hemispheres, depending on task demands. When patients are asked to point to a location, lesions in the posterior portion of both left and right hemispheres can result in deficits (Ratcliff, 1982). However, deficits of location in space, when no motor response is required, result from right hemisphere lesions (Warrington & Rabin, 1970). Subsequent studies have also supported the notion that deficits in the location in space result from right hemisphere damage and are associated with visual field defect (Hannay, Varney, & Benton, 1976).

Deficits in the direction of lines are associated with right hemisphere damage (Benton, Hamsher, Varney, & Spreen, 1983). Other studies support the idea that deficits in pure spatial perception are associated with right hemisphere lesions while deficits in tasks that require spatial rotation or orientation may be seen in left as well as right hemisphere lesions (Mehta & Newcombe, 1991).

Topographic disorientation is also more commonly associated with right than left hemisphere lesions (Landis, Cummings, Benson, & Palmer, 1986), although some deficits have been reported only in patients with bilateral parietal lobe lesions.

Deficits of depth perception and stereopsis are most reliably associated with bilateral lesions in the visual cortex, although unilateral lesions on either side can result in reduction of stereoacuity.

Visuoconstructional deficits are often referred to as constructional apraxias. Most often tests which assess these deficits require the integration of several abilities. For example, most tests of visuoconstruction require visuoperception and graphomotor abilities. As a result it is difficult to localize this ability. Some form of constructional disability is frequently present in patients with brain disease. While most studies report a slightly higher rate in unilateral right hemisphere lesions than left, any brain damaged group usually will have higher rates of constructional deficits than a control group (Benton, 1967).

Visual imagery refers to the process of recalling visual stimuli from memory stores. Some have suggested that this may be of little clinical relevance. However, in a therapeutic setting it may be important to recognize a limitation in this capacity. While normative studies have suggested that the neural pathways underlying visual imagery are similar to those that underlie visual perception, studies in patients make it difficult to determine which hemisphere is involved. Several reports indicate deficits in visual imagery in patients with left hemisphere lesions (Farah, 1984, 1986), but reinterpretation of these results suggests that both hemispheres may be involved, although in different aspects of the process (Sergent, 1990).

Impairment in facial discrimination, a very specific visuospatial ability, is twice as common with right hemisphere than left hemisphere lesions (Hamsher, Levin, & Benton, 1979), with poorest performance associated with damage to the more posterior regions. However, patients with left hemisphere posterior lesions do more poorly than controls.

Aprosodia, occurring in the absence of other aphasic disturbances, may be associated with lesions in the nondominant hemisphere. This refers to disturbances in tonal fluctuation, which occur in normal speech, often conveying emotional content through inflection. Patients with aprosodic speech may find that others are either unable to interpret their affect or misinterpret it altogether.

OTHER CONDITIONS ASSOCIATED WITH NEUROLOGICAL DAMAGE

Amnesic disorders are commonly seen in rehabilitation patients and can occur in the absence of other cognitive deficits (Drachman & Arbit, 1966). Anterograde amnesia refers to the inability to demonstrate new learning. This is sometimes referred to as recent or long-term memory deficit. The key feature is the inability to recall information that exceeds the immediate memory span. For example, the patient may be able to repeat a list of numbers or words immediately after they are presented, but would not be able to recall the information after a small delay. The inability to recall is often not improved even when multiple choice or cuing is provided. Anterograde amnesia inhibits the patient's ability to establish new memories from the time of injury and is very disabling. The memory deficit is in stark contrast to the preserved conversational languages skills, often leading the uninformed observer to have unrealistic expectations of the patient's abilities.

Retrograde amnesia refers to the loss of memory for events prior to the injury and includes loss of both factual and autobiographical information. The most common pattern of forgetting is in a temporal order with the greatest loss of those things that happened closest to the injury. However, a nontemporal loss has also been described and is usually associated with diseases such as herpes simplex encephalitis (Butters, Miliotis, Albert, & Sax, 1984; Damasio, Eslinger, Damasio, Van Hoesen, & Cornell, 1985).

Typically, amnesic patients demonstrate memory deficits across all modalities, probably because the deficit is a result of bilateral damage, as with disease or with damage to a midline structure. Modality-specific deficits have been reported in cases of lateralized lesions, with greater impairment in the recall of verbal than nonverbal material in left hemisphere lesions and the opposite pattern in right hemisphere lesions.

Achromatopsia, a disturbance of hue discrimination or the perception of grayness, can result from occipital lobe lesions. It is usually associated with a visual field defect of the superior quadrant.

Another condition seen with occipital lobe lesions is prosopagnosia, which refers to the inability to recognize a familiar face, either on a person or in a picture. This defect may extend to the inability to interpret the meaning of facial expressions. Visual field deficits are nearly always present in this condition.

Subtle sensory disturbances include extinction to double simultaneous stimulation. The extinction occurs on the contralateral side of the lesion, even though unilateral stimulation on the same side is recognized. Anosagnosia, which refers to the lack of recognition of self, is also associated with inferior parietal lobe lesions in the region of the supramarginal gyrus.

This can be manifested by ignoring grooming to one side of the body or denying somatic deficits. As some recovery occurs, patients with these lesions have been known to demonstrate catastrophic reactions, which are characterized by sudden awareness of an aspect of deficit, with distress level out of proportion to the actual deficit. Patients with dominant parietal lobe lesions without motor or sensory deficits have been found to have ideomotor apraxia. They lose the ability to perform learned motor skills on command or by imitation. For example, they may be unable to demonstrate actions such as combing hair or brushing teeth on command.

ISSUES OF NEUROPSYCHOLOGICAL ASSESSMENT

Neuropsychological assessment can play several roles for the rehabilitation patient. First, it can characterize the nature of the deficit. As illustrated above, small details of the specific deficits can make significant differences in one's ultimate disability. Second, it can identify relative strengths and weaknesses which can be used to direct the methods of rehabilitation. For example, subtle neglect can compromise one's ability to read, making reading a poor method for communicating new skills. Third, it can provide indications of premorbid function. Awareness of premorbid function is critical in setting reasonable goals for rehabilitation. Realistic expectations will permit the patient to experience success, an important motivator for maximizing the patient's participation.

There are two primary approaches to neuropsychological assessment, each with its own advantages. The first uses a standard battery of tests to systematically assess each domain. The Halstead Reitan Battery is an example of this technique. This approach makes no assumptions that any function is intact. The tests in the battery typically begin by formally assessing the sensitivity to the stimulus and to the physical ability to produce the response. Simple tasks are made more complex by adding a single demand at a time. The advantage of this thorough approach is that subtle deficits can be noted and all domains are assessed. It is of particular value in a severe extensive injury.

Another approach is to begin the assessment with more complex tasks and conduct in-depth testing of those areas which are impaired. This approach assumes that there are many different ways to accomplish a task and the focus should be on those tasks which cannot be accomplished. In this approach, the Wechsler Adult Intelligence Scale-Revised (WAIS-R) may be administered initially to determine premorbid abilities and to identify deficits which need further assessment. One can assess some levels of language comprehension and production, visuospatial abilities, and reasoning with the WAIS-R. If deficits are suggested by the pattern of performance, more detailed and structured assessment of these domains is necessary. Additional testing of domains not tapped by the WAIS-R must also be included. The advantage of this approach is that it evaluates cognition as a whole, identifying problems with accomplishing tasks that may more closely approximate functional abilities. It may eliminate testing of unnecessary domains.

The other areas which are important to assess include attention and concentration, memory and learning, concept formation and abstract reasoning, verbal and language functions including reading and naming, and speed of information processing. These areas are particularly important in milder forms of injury or after recovery from gross neurological and neuropsychological deficits. There is a wide choice of tests for assessing each domain (for a review of tests, their application, and available normative data see Lezak [1995]). It is important to acknowledge that most neuropsychological tests are complex and examine more than one function. For this reason, poor performance in any test must be explored to isolate which function is actually impaired. Selection may be based on the normative data available for a given measure as well as the ability of a test to meet the specific needs of a particular patient. For example, assessment of visual memory or attention in a patient with a hemiparesis would avoid tests which require constructions or other graphomotor responses.

The neuropsychological report will often attempt to attribute performance to injury or premorbid factors. While this is never done with complete certainty, there are profiles of performance which are associated with noninjury factors.When these factors are part of the clinical history, it is important to weigh their impact on cognitive performance. For example, a history of learning disability, alcohol use, or major depression can be associated with cognitive deficits. In the case of stroke, diseases of aging, including prior stroke or preexisting cognitive decline, may also be considered. In a conservative approach to the assessment, deficits associated with the premorbid condition would be acknowledged and only residual deficits could be attributed to the injury. In some cases the severity of a deficit may indicate contributions from several factors.

AFFECTIVE DISTURBANCES AND NEUROPSYCHOLOGICAL DEFICITS

Patients with brain injury often have changes in emotional experience and behavior. The expression of an appropriate emotion may depend in part on the ability to comprehend emotional stimuli. As mentioned above, many patients with brain injury have difficulty comprehending the visual stimuli which express emotions, with poorest performance from those with right brain injury. In general, the deficits seen in right brain injury are not valence dependent and are not emotion specific (Borod, Koff, Perlman-Lorch, & Nicholas, 1986). Patients with right brain damage also have trouble comprehending some of the vocal nuances that convey emotion in speech (Heilman, Bowers, Speedie, & Coslett, 1984). Some authors have found that the facial expression of emotion is reduced in patients with right hemisphere brain injury, although this is not consistently reported. There is substantial evidence that lesions of the frontal lobe are critical to the reduction of emotional facial expression, regardless of which side.

    Another aspect of the effect of the lesion is the experience of emotion. It has been reported that patients with right hemisphere disease appear to be euphoric or indifferent, while several studies have suggested that left hemisphere lesions are associated with depression. The depressive syndrome is usually seen in nonfluent aphasics with lesions in the anterior regions of the frontal lobe. It can also be seen in patients with subcortical injury. The severity of the depression seems to increase with proximity to the frontal pole (Starkstein, Robinson, & Price, 1987) and is characterized by the presence of significant anxiety. More recent studies have suggested that right hemisphere patients also experience a high level of depression, but it goes undetected because of their difficulty with emotional expression (House, Dennis, Warlow, Hawton, & Molyneux, 1990).

Other aberrations of emotional expression can be seen in patients with limbic system involvement. Both animal lesion studies and human observational studies lead to a complex story of the role of the limbic system in emotion. However, it is important to note that brain lesions can produce rage (Zeman & King, 1958), placidity (Poeck, 1969), aggression (Pincus, 1980), fear and anxiety (Strauss, Risser, & Jones, 1982), hyposexuality (Taylor, 1969), and increased libido (Cogen, Antunes, & Correll, 1979).

DEFICITS IN MILD HEAD INJURY

Patients with spinal cord injuries may also have mild traumatic brain injury (MTBI), with estimates ranging from 40 to 50% (Davidoff et al., 1992). Mild traumatic brain injury is defined by the presence of a subtle cognitive disturbance consisting of one of the following: (1) brief (less than 30 minutes) period of loss of consciousness; (2) loss of memory for events before or after the injury; (3) altered mental states (often reported as "dazed, disoriented, or confused"); and (4) transient or persistent focal neurological deficit. These deficits can occur with a blow to the head or an acceleration–deceleration (e.g., whiplash) injury. In the face of serious spinal cord injury, the possibility of MTBI may be overlooked. However, this entity can be associated with symptoms which can impede rehabilitation efforts.

Three broad categories of symptoms are noted with MTBI. The physical symptoms include nausea and vomiting, which are most common immediately after the injury. Other symptoms which may persist include dizziness, blurred vision, sleep disturbance, fatigue, and sensory disturbance. Cognitive difficulties include problems with attention, concentration, perception, minor speech and language deficits, and executive (i.e., planning) deficits. These deficits may be so subtle that they are difficult to capture in formal testing. Behavioral symptoms include anger, irritability, changes in emotional responsiveness, disinhibition, and emotional lability.

These symptoms and complaints may be particularly problematic in a patient in the rehabilitation setting. They can interfere with ability to benefit from rehabilitation. It is usually assumed that these symptoms are most prominent immediately after the accident with significant recovery over time. It is estimated that 60 to 90% of patients with MTBI recover within a year. However, there is persistence of these symptoms in the first 3 to 6 months, which is usually the interval when patients with acute injuries are participating in rehabilitation. The cognitive symptoms may not even become evident until rehabilitation begins, because this reflects the first challenge to these skills. It may be difficult to determine the etiology of these symptoms. In fact, multiple musculoskeletal injuries, which may occur in serious accidents as well as in minor injuries, can produce many of the same physical symptoms and complaints associated with MTBI. For example, in the absence of spinal cord injury, soft tissue injury can cause disturbances of sensation, including tingling or burning sensations. Chronic muscle pain may be associated with fatigue and increased irritability. Musculoskeletal injuries of the neck and shoulders can be associated with headache and complaints of blurred vision. It is therefore important to carefully consider the range of possible etiologies including brain injury when developing a plan for recovery.

OTHER PHYSICAL DISTURBANCES

Traumatic brain injury (TBI) can produce dysfunctional sensations. These include visual field defects that can be compensated for by increased concentration and neck motion. There can be alterations in sensation of vibration, temperature, position sense, light touch, and pain. These altered sensations produce physical challenges by decreasing awareness of the environment which can lead to falls, injuries, and skin breakdown. Damage to the cranial nerves can cause diplopia, blurred vision, nystagmus, dizziness, hearing impairment, facial paralysis, decreased taste and smell, and dysarthria. Visual field deficits can cause difficulties with the activities of daily living, the patient's driving, and employment.

Spasticity produces frequent physical challenges for patients with spinal cord and traumatic brain injury. It is a difficult problem to treat. Drugs that reduce spasticity frequently produce fatigue and lack of coordination. Chronic spasticity can progressively limit joint range of motion and produce flexion contractures. The flexion contractures are painful and further reduce the patient's mobility and independence. Management of spasticity involves active and passive exercises. These help to decrease the spasticity for a period of time and help preserve the range of motion. Bracing can help to prevent spasticity and can also be useful to help correct joint deformities. Surgery has also been used and has been most successful in treating spasticity in the lower extremities.

PHYSICAL CHALLENGES AND ISSUES OF DISABILITY

Patients will have increased functional challenges the higher the level of the spinal cord injury. Patients with lesions from the C2 to C7 will require assistance with routine urinary catheterization and bowel routine. With lesions at the C2 to 3 level, the patient will be totally dependent in activities of daily living and be respirator dependent. A phrenic nerve pacemaker may allow some patients to avoid respirator dependence. A patient with a lesion at the C-4 level will still be dependent in activities of daily living and transferring. However, they may have some mobility by using a powered wheelchair with a chin control, or a sip and puff control unit. Patients with lesions at the C-5 level are able to self-feed and brush their teeth with assistive devices.

They may also drive a powered wheelchair with a hand-control unit. Patients with lesions at the C-6 level can push a manual wheelchair with vertical tips on the hand rims. They have potential independence in self-care activities, and can be independent in transferring from bed to wheelchair using a sliding board. They may be able to drive a van with hand controls and power door lift. With the C-7 level lesion, self-care activities are much easier and a manual wheelchair will be sufficient for locomotion. Patients with C-8 to T-1 level lesions can have full independence although they will be wheelchair bound. In lesions at the T-2 through L-3 level, the paralyzed individual will be completely independent and wheelchair bound, and have better stamina because of minimal respiratory and upper extremity limitations. L4 to 5 paraplegics are able to walk with leg braces and crutches. S-1 level paralysis will require braces and crutches, and because of the neurogenic bladder and bowel, require intermittent catheterization and a regular bowel program.

PHYSICAL CHALLENGES ASSOCIATED WITH BRAIN INJURY

Patients with brain injury often have unilateral impairment which may permit them to compensate for physical limitations with their unaffected side. However, they frequently have trouble with activities of daily living because of their unique neurological impairment. Patients with brain injury can have impairments in one or more physical functions which will impair their feeding skills. Dysphagia, difficulty swallowing, is commonly seen in patients with brain injury and may result in dietary restrictions. These patients are at a greater risk for aspirating with thin liquids than thick liquids. Food consumption may be limited to pureed, soft, minced, or regular food. Impairments in feeding may also result from hemiparesis, contractures, spasticity, sensory deficits, poor head control, and impaired balance. These patients may need help with feeding and/or assistive devices such as positioning aides, splints, or adaptive utensils. Cognitive and perceptual deficits may impede the progress of learning to incorporate assistive devices. For example, patients with neglect may leave food in one side of their mouth. This neglect can lead to aspiration.

The ability to dress and complete hygiene skills can be compromised in the head injured patient. Hemiparesis or hemiplegia may impede these activities. In addition, visual neglect, anasanosia, and apraxias can further limit the accomplishment of these functional activities. Specific training with adaptive aides and bathroom modifications such as bath bars, raised toilet seats, and shower chairs may be helpful. These patients may also need to have a routine set up for them, which will organize the activity and require minimal initiation on their part.

Communication skills may be severely impaired following brain injury. Aphasia, alexia, agraphia all contribute to the patient's inability to write, type, or use the telephone. Adaptive aides may be useful when neglect, weakness, visual field cut, or incoordination are the source of the problems.

Homemaking skills present a series of physical challenges to patients with brain injury. Physical limitations may reduce independence in cooking and cleaning. Decreased sensation or neglect can cause serious burns in patients because of lack of awareness of potentially dangerous situations. Cognitive problems, such as impulse control, difficulties with judgment and problem solving abilities, can also increase the risk of unsafe behavior in homemaking activities. Both physical ability and safety must be considered when determining one's ability to perform independently. In some cases, maximum independence will always require supervision to perform homemaking tasks.

There are many aspects to the challenge of mobility outside the home for patients with brain injury. Driving can be impaired by seizures, visual field defects, or neglect. Medications can cause drowsiness. Poor judgment can make driving unsafe. While adaptive devices can permit driving in the presence of motor weakness, they do require intact perception and judgment.

Other independent living skills also offer physical challenges, such as shopping and recreation. Shopping involves the recognition of need, the organization of transportation for the activity, selection of items, and management of money. Patients with brain injury may have problems with all or any of these areas. Because of physical limitations prohibiting driving, many times these patients will need to use public transportation. Strategies for these activities include getting on and off at the same stop, and carrying fare in the same place, which help to eliminate confusion. Patients will have difficulty with recreational activities, and may need to find new hobbies or activities they can perform that are within their new limitations.

MEETING THE CHALLENGE IN THE FACE OF PREMORBID FACTORS

Identification of premorbid conditions is an important step in understanding how the patient will meet the physical challenges facing them. Patients with a traumatic injury often have a preexisting history of learning disability, substance abuse, prior arrests and incarcerations, and psychological problems including personality disorders (Fahy, Irving, & Millag, 1967; Rosenthal & Bond, 1990). Alternately, brain injury may reflect an event over which a patient had no control and premorbid characteristics and self-perceptions may play a role in the ability to rise to the challenges that occur. Patients with stroke may have had a previous stroke, or other unaddressed risk factors including uncontrolled hypertension or diabetes. A history of all aspects of the patient's life may be needed and many sources may be called on to accomplish this, including family members, employers, school records, teachers, and friends. Family members can often provide information, but it may be biased by fear that negative information about the patient may alienate the staff, inadvertently set a low expectation for recovery, or jeopardize a legal claim. Consequently, it is important to get a broad view of the patient's premorbid status.

Since many patients will have increased dependence on others after the injury, it is important to understand the dynamics of their interpersonal relationships. In the case of a patient who will return to a home setting, preexisting tensions between the patient and the family will interfere with their ability to provide the appropriate level of supervision and independence.

Preexisting substance abuse, a not uncommon condition in traumatic injury (Heinemann, Keen, Donohue, & Schnoll, 1988), is unlikely to resolve without intervention. This is true of noncompliance with medical treatments for conditions such as diabetes or hypertension, which increase the risk of stroke. While these may be controlled in the rehabilitation setting, in a less restrictive environment, these patterns are likely to return. In the patient who faces physical challenges because of their injury, the use of drugs or alcohol has a heightened likelihood of causing reckless behavior and reinjury.

Psychological factors often contribute to the behavior that led a patient to the injury. These factors must be addressed to maximize the patient's new limitations and to avoid returning to high-risk behavior.

The return to employment is part of a rehabilitation assessment. However, the work setting often provides a set of physical challenges. If return to work is part of the goal, one must assess premorbid employment history. Both the type of job and the work habits need to be addressed. The simplest reentry to employment would be to return to a preinjury job. This may require adaptations to the workplace, assistive devices, and flexible hours. It may not be possible to adapt some jobs, particularly if they involve intense physical labor. Retraining for more sedentary positions may be desirable, but premorbid educational level and academic history may limit the potential for retraining. The neuropsychological deficits of the present accident must also be considered when retraining is being proposed.

CONCLUSIONS

There is a wide range of cognitive deficits and physical challenges experienced by patients in the rehabilitation setting.

Acknowledging the breadth of these problems permits one to develop realistic goals for recovery. Injury usually impacts on many aspects of the nervous system and many functions and behaviors are controlled to a greater or lesser degree by several different brain locations. Therefore, it is unlikely that a single description will capture the nuances experienced by an individual. However, understanding the most probable patterns of deficit may provide a schema within which to approach the patient.

REFERENCES

Behrmann, M., Moskovitch, M., Black, S. E., & Mozer, M. (1990). Perceptual and conceptual mechanisms in neglect dyslexia. *Brain, 113,* 1163–1183.

Benson, D. F. (1979). *Aphasia, alexia and agraphia.* New York: Churchill Livingston.

Benton, A. L. (1967). Constructional apraxia and the minor hemisphere. *Confinia Neurologica, 29,* 1–16.

Benton, A. L., Hamsher, K., Varney, N. R., & Spreen, O. (1983). *Contributions to neuropsychological assessment.* New York: Oxford University Press.

Borod, J., Koff, E., Perlman-Lorch, J., & Nicholas, M. (1986). The expression and perception of facial emotions in brain damaged patients. *Neuropsychologia, 24,* 169–180.

Butters, N., Miliotis, P., Albert, M. D., & Sax, D. S. (1984). Memory assessment: Evidence of the heterogeneity of amnesic symptoms. In G. Goldstein (Ed.), *Advances in clinical neuropsychology* (Vol. 1); pp. 127–159). New York: Plenum.

Cogen, P. H., Antunes, J. L., & Correll, J. W. (1979). Reproductive function in temporal lobe epilepsy: The effect of temporal lobe lobectomy. *Surgical Neurology, 12,* 243–246.

Damasio, A. R., Eslinger, P. J., Damasio, H., Van Hoesen, G. W., & Cornell, S. (1985). Multimodal amnesic syndrome following bilateral temporal and basal forebrain damage. *Archives of Neurology, 42,* 252–259.

Davidoff, G. N., Roth, E. J., & Richards, S. (1992). Cognitive deficits in spinal cord injury: Epidemiology and outcome. *Archives of Physical Medicine and Rehabilitation, 73,* 375–384.

De Renzi, E., & Spinnler, H. (1967). Impaired performance on color tasks in patients with hemispheric damage. *Cortex, 3,* 194–216.

Drachman, D. A., & Arbit, J. (1966). Memory and the hippocampal complex. *Archives of Neurology, 15,* 52–61.

Fahy, T. J., Irving, M. H., & Millag, P. (1967). Severe head injuries: A six year follow-up. *Lancet, 2,* 475.

Farah, M. J. (1984). The neurological basis of mental imagery: A componential analysis. *Cognition, 18,* 245–272.

Farah, M. J. (1986). The laterality of mental image generation: A test with normal subjects. *Neuropsychologia, 24,* 541–551.

Frankel, H. L. (1969). The value of postural reduction in the initial management of closed injuries of spine with paraplegia and tetraplegia: Comprehensive management and research. *Paraplegia, 7,* 179.

Hamsher, K., Levin, H. S., & Benton, A. L. (1979). Facial recognition in patients with focal brain lesions. *Archives of Neurology, 36,* 837–839.

Hannay, H. J., Varney, N. R., & Benton, A. L. (1976). Visual localization in patients with unilateral brain disease. *Journal of Neurology, Neurosurgery, and Psychiatry, 39,* 307–313.

Hecaen, H., & Albert, M. L. (1978). *Human neuropsychology.* New York: Wiley.

Heilman, K. M., Bowers, D., Speedie, L., & Coslett, B. (1984). Comprehension of affective and nonaffective speech. *Neurology, 34,* 917–921.

Heinemann, A. W., Keen, M., Donohue, R., & Schnoll, S. (1988). Alcohol use in persons with recent spinal cord injuries. *Archives of Physical Medicine and Rehabilitation, 69,* 619–624.

House, A., Dennis, M., Warlow, C., Hawton, K., & Molyneux, A. (1990). Mood disorders after stroke and their relation to lesion location. *Brain, 113,* 1113–1129.

Kinsbourne, M., & Warrington, E. K. (1962). A variety of reading disability associated with right hemisphere lesions. *Journal of Neurology, Neurosurgery and Psychiatry, 25,* 339–344.

Landis, T., Cummings, J. L., Benson, D. F., & Palmer, E. P. (1986). Loss of topographic familiarity: An environmental agnosia. *Archives of Neurology, 43,* 132–136.

Lezak, M. D. (1995). *Neuropsychological assessment* (3rd ed.). New York: Oxford University Press.

Mehta, Z., & Newcombe, F. (1991). A role for the left hemisphere in spatial processing. *Cortex, 27,* 153–167.

Pincus, J. H. (1980). Can violence be a manifestation of epilepsy? *Neurology, 30,* 304–307.

Poeck, K. (1969). Pathophysiology of emotional disorders associated with brain damage. In P. J. Vinken & G. W. Bruyn (Eds.), *Handbook of neurology* (Vol. 3; pp. 343–367). New York: Elsevier.

Ratcliff, G. (1982). Disturbances of spatial orientation associated with cerebral lesions. In M. Potegal (Ed.), *Spatial abilities: Development and physiological foundations* (pp. 301–333). New York: Academic.

Rosenthal, M., & Bond, M. (1990). Behavioral and psychiatric sequelae. In M. Rosenthal, E. Griffith, M. Bond, & J. Miller (Eds.), *Rehabilitation of the adult and child with traumatic brain injury* (2nd ed.; pp. 179–192). Philadelphia: F. A. Davis.

Sergent, J. (1990). The neuropsychology of visual image generation: Data, method and theory. *Brain and Cognition, 13*, 98–129.

Starkstein, S. E., Robinson, R. G., & Price, T. R. (1987). Comparison of cortical and subcortical lesions in the production of poststroke mood disorders. *Brain, 110*, 1045–1059.

Strauss, E., Risser, A., & Jones, M. W. (1982). Fear responses in patients with epilepsy. *Neurology, 39*, 626–630.

Taylor, D. C. (1969). Aggression and epilepsy. *Journal of Psychiatric Research, 13*, 229–236.

Warrington, E. K., & Rabin, P. (1970). Perceptual matching in patients with cerebral lesions. *Neuropsychologia, 8*, 475–487.

Zeman, W., & King, F. A. (1958). Tumors of the septum pellucidum and adjacent structures with abnormal affective behavior: An anterior midline structure syndrome. *Journal of Nervous and Mental Disorders, 127*, 490–502.

2.

A History of Psychotherapy with Patients with Brain Injury

Laurence Miller, Ph.D.

As recently as a week prior to this writing, a neurologist colleague, upon hearing that I was preparing a chapter on psychotherapy with patients with brain injury, queried bluntly, "What the hell can you do for those people?"

"What we do for" our patients with organic brain syndromes is the subject of this volume, and to know where we're going, it's useful to know where we've been. Most of the conceptual confusion and clinical public relations difficulties in advocating psychotherapy as a legitimate, indeed vital, aspect of brain injury rehabilitation comes from the entrenched, traditional dichotomy of *organic* vs. *psychological.* Neuromedical research is pinning down psychological symptoms to PET-enhanced cerebral structures, and physicians routinely take double board certification in neurology and psychiatry. But even in the late 1990s there persists a clinical mindset that is apparently more willing to accept a biological component for depression or psychosis, than a psychodynamic dimension to the adaptive recovery from acquired brain injury.

The history in this chapter is a dual one, because neuropsychology and psychodynamics have always nourished one another—indeed, one could not exist without the other (Miller,

1991, 1997, 1998b, in press). This chapter will provide a conceptual history of psychotherapeutic approaches that have recognized this important link. The focus will be on one important meeting ground between the two disciplines, namely *cognition*. As human beings are thinking creatures, the vagaries of cognition, along with its sister functions, emotion and action, lie at the very core of the concept of *selfhood*. And it is this shattered self that effective psychotherapy with patients who are neuropsychologically impaired must fundamentally address (Miller, 1993a, 1998a).

THE ORGANIC PERSONALITY

Neuropsychologists know that there are many individual variations of the clinical picture seen after brain damage, depending on the type and location of the injury, as well as the patient's preexisting and predisposing characteristics. However, certain behavioral commonalities are typically found in brain injured patients as a whole. Historically, one of the first and best comprehensive descriptions of the *organic personality* as a unitary, composite, clinical entity comes from the work of Kurt Goldstein (1952). Goldstein (1952) conceived of brain damage as impairing the person's ability to make the necessary adaptations to his or her world in the service of discharging tensions and satisfying needs—what psychoanalytic clinicians like Hartmann (1939/1958) were calling *adaptive ego functions*.

Thus, observed Goldstein (1952), some organically impaired patients are unable to bear even small changes in environment or routine. Others cannot sustain close relationships because this usually involves tolerating some degree of frustration of immediate needs. Such patients may appear overly demanding, clingy, or "childish." Still others can't cope with the disability caused by the brain damage, and its effect on their lives.

Many such patients learn to achieve a kind of fragile equilibrium, wherein they constrain their range of activities in different environments to a level that their altered cognitive capacities can handle. This, Goldstein (1952) pointed out, often requires nothing less than a redefinition of the person's identity and self-image. This is difficult enough for a physically disabled person with an otherwise intact brain, but a colossal undertaking for someone who has sustained an injury to the very organ of adaptation itself.

Aside from focal deficits such as aphasias, aprosodias, apraxias, agnosias, and amnesias, much of the difficulties experienced by the patient who has brain injury were attributed by Goldstein (1952; Goldstein & Scheerer, 1941) to what he called a *loss of the abstract attitude*. Although seen most often in patients with frontal lobe damage, it also occurs frequently in many other kinds of focal or generalized brain injury. This is not surprising, as Goldstein pointed out, since the frontal lobes constitute about one-third of the entire human brain volume, so sufficient impact anywhere in the cranium is bound to affect the frontal region to some degree.

It is this abstract attitude, said Goldstein (1952; Goldstein & Scheerer, 1941), that enables a person to flexibly detach their ego from the outer world or inner experience. It enables us to assume a particular mental set, to account to oneself for one's own behavior and to verbalize that account. It enables us to shift reflectively from one aspect of a situation to another, to hold several aspects of a situation or problem in mind simultaneously, and to grasp the essentials of a given whole. We can break up a given whole into parts, and isolate and synthesize these parts. We can abstract common properties of a thing reflectively and form hierarchic concepts. We are enabled to plan ahead ideationally, to assume an attitude toward the "mere possible," and to think or perform symbolically.

Luria (1973, 1980), who cited Goldstein's work extensively (and, to a lesser extent, Freud's), subsequently conducted his now classic studies of the neuropsychology of cognition, and outlined the stages ordinarily involved in what we regard as mature, productive thought. First, there must exist a task or problem for which there is no instinctual or automatically habitual solution. Next, there must be some motivation for solving that problem. Further, the person must be able to restrain

impulsive responding, and be capable of investigating and analyzing the features of the problem. Out of many possible alternative courses of action, the individual must select those few
that are judged to be most appropriate, sequence the action
appropriately, then put the plan into effect, and finally, evaluate the results against the original goal. This automatic cognitive cascade is what largely facilitates mature, adult, adaptive
thought and behavior.

When the adaptive capacity of the individual is strained to
the breaking point—which happens all too frequently for the
brain injured individual—the clinician may observe what
Goldstein (1952) characterized as the *catastrophic reaction*. Expressions of this decompensation may range from the frankly
explosive—the patient screams, curses, lashes out, throws
things—to more subtle and therefore more easily overlooked
manifestations, such as passive withdrawal, regression, smolder-
ing hostility, sullen refusal to cooperate, or failure to participate in self-care.

Over time, said Goldstein (1952), the patient with a brain
injury begins to develop *protective mechanisms* in order to forestall anxiety, frustration, and the catastrophic reaction. Examples of this include denial of deficit and withdrawal from
demanding and frustrating activities. The latter frequently
plays havoc with rehabilitation staff, who may not understand
why the patient "doesn't want to get better," insufficiently ap-
preciating what a blow to self-esteem and self-image each little
failure and struggle entails. Obsessive–compulsive behavior
may develop as the patient tries to achieve maximal control
over a delimited aspect of his or her environment.

An inability to fully comprehend the requirements of the
social milieu may lead to a variety of "immature" or "inappropriate" behaviors. The need to discharge tension immediately
may be expressed in impulsive, angry, and "entitled" demands
for food, cigarettes, sex, privileges, and so on. The concreteness
associated with neurocognitive impairment may lead to a
"coarsening" of thought, feeling, and action, as well as a loss
of the patient's sense of humor.

More recently, Lewis and Rosenberg (1990), drawing on their experience with patients who have traumatic head injuries, have presented a characterization of the "organic personality" that comes close to the one offered earlier by Goldstein (1952). Patients with brain injury, in this account, must struggle with high levels of anxiety at the same time that their capacity to tolerate painful emotions of any type has been reduced. Heightened affective arousal, coupled with reduced tolerance of affect, is a perfect set-up for the appearance of catastrophic reactions and other forms of decompensation. By virtue of the neurologic dysfunction and resultant cognitive deficits, the patient is less adept at smoothly integrating raw feeling with refined perceptual apprehension and cognitive understanding.

The brain injury has thus created a condition that Lewis, Allen, and Frieswyk (1983) call *cortical vulnerability:* These patients tolerate emotion poorly because brain damage has deprived them of the capacity to sufficiently titrate and modulate emotion in a way that makes it comprehensible and manageable. This may be exacerbated by a tendency to actively avoid thinking about, or "dwelling on," painful feelings, thereby precluding the development of adaptive coping—an attitude often abetted by well-meaning persons seeking to avoid "upsetting" the patient.

Yet other patients, even without a history of acquired brain injury, seem to encounter "upsetting" situations all too frequently, and to characteristically cope with them poorly. What has neuropsychology and psychodynamic theory had to offer these patients?

THE PRIMITIVE PERSONALITY

The psychodynamic side of this chapter's history begins, appropriately enough, with Freud. Freud (1900/1953, 1915/1957, 1923/1961) originally proposed that the transformation of primitive instinctual impulses into consciously acceptable substitutive drive derivatives utilizes the cognitive processes of symbolization and language. The purpose of thinking, said Freud, is to permit the ego to achieve a delay of motor discharge, to serve as a kind of "experimental action" which allows for the exploration of behavioral alternatives with far less effort and painful consequence than would be required for the real-world testing of each different alternative.

But Freud failed to elaborate on the roles of these cognitive processes in the development of personality, preferring to concentrate on the role of instinct. It became the task of the later ego psychologists, exemplified by Heinz Hartmann (1939/1958), to stress the importance of what they regarded as constitutionally given mental endowments and apparatuses for psychological development—such faculties as memory, perception, attention, and intelligence. According to Hartmann (1939/1958), these basic human adaptive apparatuses comprise a core of adaptive psychological functioning that is relatively independent of instinctual conflict, constituting the *conflict-free ego sphere.* These apparatuses also influence the different ways of handling conflict; that is, they are the underpinnings of the classic psychological defenses.

Hartmann (1939/1958) proposed that evolution leads to increasing independence of the organism from its environment so that reactions which originally occurred in relation to the external world are progressively displaced to the interior of the organism, that is, to a mental domain. In order to achieve a certain adaptation to and mastery of the world, a person need not test every possible response and observe every possible reaction. Rather, he or she can think about consequences, anticipate outcomes, and create contingency plans of alternative means–end possibilities, which Hartmann collectively described as the process of *internalization.* Accordingly, Hartmann spoke of *ego autonomy* as involving the relative freedom of the ego or self from blind obediance to instinctual emotional and motivational demands, as well as from a dependency on immediate environmental reinforcement for each action and plan.

The term *cognitive style* was introduced by George S. Klein (1954, 1958) to refer to the arrangement of general regulatory or control structures in each person's psyche, having their basis in the constitutional faculties suggested by Hartmann (1939/

1958). An unfortunately little-known and underappreciated research project was carried out by Gardner, Holzman, Klein, Linton, and Spence (1959) which explored the relationship between psychodynamics, cognitive style, and psychopathology, and served historically as the foundation of many of the "projective tests" routinely used by psychoanalytically oriented clinicians (Rapaport, Gill, & Schafer, 1968). David Shapiro (1965) subsequently used the term *style* in his conceptualization of *neurotic styles;* i.e., characteristic maladaptive modes of functioning that are built around each person's characterological style of perception, thought, and action.

Symptoms or prominent pathological traits, said Shapiro (1965), regularly appear in the context of attitudes, interests, intellectual inclinations and endowments, and even vocational aptitudes and social affinities with which the given symptom or trait seems to have a certain consistency. Accordingly, neurosis is not simply the result of instinctually driven, intrapsychic conflict superimposed on a tabula rasa personality. Rather, the form that the neurotic expression of conflict takes is strongly determined by how that person perceives the world, thinks about it, reacts emotionally to it, and behaves in it; that is, by how his or her own set of constitutional cognitive traits is arrayed in the psyche. Shapiro (1965) identified four main neurotic styles: the obsessive–compulsive, the paranoid, the hysterical, and the impulsive, providing the foundation for a later neuropsychodynamic conceptualization of personality by Miller (1990, 1991).

More recently, Shapiro (1989) has asserted that the neurotic patient is "estranged from himself" to the extent that his maladaptive or neurotic cognitive style contributes to the obfuscation of his own motivations and interpretations of external reality. Shapiro's (1989) neurotic personality is reminiscent of Goldstein's (1952) descriptions of the organic personality and Luria's (1973, 1980) studies of frontal lobe deficits in verbal self-regulation. Shapiro's (1989) neurotic personality reacts not deliberatively, proactively, and autonomously, but rather quasireflexively to dispel or forestall external anxiety or internal psychical discomfort produced by self-perceptions that threaten the all too brittle and fragile stability of the personality structure.

Robbins (1989) has provided a description of the *primitive personality*, under which he subsumes the borderline, narcissistic, paranoid, and schizoid personality types. Other writers have also included the impulsive and hysterical personalities in this category (Begun, 1976; Masterson, 1988; Millon, 1981, 1990; Shapiro, 1965). The key feature of primitive personalities is the fundamentally compromised, non-self-aware, poorly self-regulated, and often self-destructive existences these individuals typically lead.

Primitive personalities show deficient personality integration, being characteristically dominated by self-contradictory thinking. Their emotional life is typically undifferentiated from raw perception and nonreflective action. Like children, or some neuropsychologically impaired individuals, primitive personalities tend to be concretely immersed in their immediate interpersonal surroundings. They misconstrue their own cognitive–affective conceptualizations of others, and experience strong urges to act impulsively toward these persons in a possessive, controlling, destructive, or distancing manner. Finally, primitive personalities suffer from an inability to identify and sustain core emotions, leading to affective lability and unstable emotional attachments.

Thus, the synchronies between patients whose adaptive capacities have been shattered by acquired brain injury—not to mention those in which these capacities never fully developed because of impaired neuropsychodevelopment—are therefore obvious. Consequently, the treatment considerations may share a similar correspondence.

COGNITIVE REHABILITATION AND PSYCHOTHERAPY WITH THE ORGANIC PATIENT

Goldstein's (1952; Goldstein & Scheerer, 1941) and Luria's (1973, 1980) neuropsychodynamic conceptualization of organic brain syndromes have begun to find practical application in the neuropsychologically informed psychotherapeutic approaches that are being developed in treatment centers throughout the country, and that form the subject matter of the present volume. Much of the impetus for developing more refined and comprehensive psychotherapeutic approaches for patients with brain injury has emerged from clinicians' and patients' frustration with the oversimple, even puerile, quality of some of the materials used in so-called "cognitive rehabilitation." In addition there is the saturation effect of continued and tedious practice of gamelike computer programs, with little attention to emotional and psychosocial issues (Carberry & Burd, 1985, 1986). Even "behavioral self-management," with its empowering-sounding connotations, often boils down to the robotic repetition and arbitrary enforcement of behavioral rules and routines. As some neurorehabilitation practitioners (Ben-Yishay & Diller, 1983, 1993) have pointed out, rehabilitation efforts which emphasize cognition and behavior, to the neglect of emotion and selfhood, omit the important function of helping the patient in his attempt to redefine and integrate a new identity.

Historically, the work of Leonard Small (1973, 1980) marked a major turning point in moving neuropsychology from its predominant focus on psychometric assessment and localization of function to an emphasis on psychodynamically informed diagnosis and in-depth psychotherapeutic treatment of a variety of organic brain syndromes. Small (1980) pointed out that brain damage often results in behavioral regression, due in large part to the dissolution of higher integrative cognitive skills necessary for complex adaptational tasks. Even as recovery and improvement in cognitive functioning occur, the patient may cling to more regressed modes of functioning because they have become predictable and manageable. Careful encouragement, support, and step-by-step training may be necessary to enable such a patient to utilize his or her recovering capacities. Forcing a too early renunciation of "immature" defenses and coping patterns may precipitate a catastrophic reaction and instill massive resistance to further therapeutic progress.

Denial, said Small (1980), especially when severe and pervasive, is probably the most difficult of the defenses to deal with, and organic denial is often refractory to any kind of psychotherapeutic approach. In other cases, denial serves a more psychodynamically based, ego-protective function which, however, may be maladaptive because it prevents the development of a realistic self-concept and impedes efforts to focus on areas where true progress can be made. The approach, then, should be not so much a confrontation or challenge, but rather a gradual focus on reality that continually monitors the patient's ego tolerance as it proceeds. Partial insights and interpretations should take precedence over ultimate ones, so that sufficient time is allowed for a reaction to the partial interpretation to be elaborated and judged.

Another pioneer in the psychotherapy of patients with brain injury has been George Prigatano (1991; Prigatano et al., 1986) whose work clearly recognizes that cognitive and emotional issues are rarely separable in the real clinical world of brain injury. Prigatano et al. (1986) point out that when patients are cognitively confused, they are generally not clear about what their feeling states are. When the confusion subsides, feelings of depression and deep sorrow often emerge. Also, many of the interpersonal problems that a person with brain injury experiences are related to faulty thinking and incorrect assumptions he or she may make about him- or herself in certain situations. There is also a tendency for patients with brain injury to deny and cover up deficits by increased rigidity of thinking. Interpersonal dialogue is thus often characterized by cognitive rigidity, loose associations, missing the main point, tunnel vision, and egocentricity. Prigatano et al.'s (1986) development of group therapy approaches to foster self-reflective psychosocial adaptation has become a model replicated around the world.

More recent contributions to psychodynamically oriented psychotherapy with patients who have a brain injury include that of Lisa Lewis and her colleagues (Lewis & Rosenberg, 1990; Lewis et al., 1983), who emphasize the effects of patients' premorbid personalities in determining whether therapy and the therapist are seen as a benefit, or as a threat and a burden.

Patients whose preexisting level of ego organization is in the borderline range probably never fully developed the capacity to use adaptive ideation and self-reflection in the first place. In psychotherapy they are encouraged to reflect on their experiences, and therapy quickly becomes an onerous chore, as their ability to use thinking in the service of self-understanding, problem solving, and planning a course of adaptive behavior—vestigial at best, even before the brain injury—are challenged.

Psychotherapy, with its thrust toward growth and autonomy, may thus be viewed by such patients with considerable ambivalence. Also, patients may be reluctant to make changes that are genuinely within their capacity for fear that others will perceive them as more competent, or less impaired, than they actually are, and then abandon them. Further, patients with brain injury are sometimes plagued by guilt, with the injury perceived as just punishment. Psychotherapy, with its implicit promise of a fuller and more productive life, may therefore be viewed negatively, and the patient's feelings of guilt and "badness" must therefore be directly addressed. Many such patients, therefore, show marked "resistance," and the therapist must then continually tread the fine line between stimulating the patient's latent capacities for adaptive thought and action, and pushing the patient beyond his or her limits, thereby creating the set-up for a catastrophic reaction.

Similarly, the work of Karen Langer (1992) explicates the diverse varieties of emotional syndromes, psychological reactions, and distortions of personality that may both follow and underlie a patient's response to brain injury. Her work teaches us never to forget the individuality of each patient's neuropsychodynamics in planning and implementing effective psychotherapeutic and rehabilitative strategies.

PSYCHOTHERAPY, PERSONALITY, AND COGNITIVE STYLE

But it works the other way, too. If the line between rehabilitation and psychotherapy is a fluid one in the case of brain injured patients, it is all the more so for patients with "primitive" personalities, often overlapping with those described as having neurotic cognitive styles (Shapiro, 1965). The term *neurotic* is understood by some psychodynamic theorists to signify a somewhat higher level of ego integration than "personality disorder," or "character pathology."

According to Erickson and Burton (1986), the kind of cognitive impairment relevant to overall rehabilitation of psychiatric and other psychotherapy patients seldom consists of discrete deficits specifically associated with brain damage, such as aphasias, apraxias, or visual field defects. Rather, they typically represent more general deficiencies in higher level complex processes such as attention and concentration, learning and memory, psychomotor speed, and problem solving. Such deficiencies are not only found among patients with brain injury and chronic psychiatric patients, but may also occur with normal aging, various personality disorders, and substance abuse.

Robbins (1989) speaks about the difficulty frequently encountered by clinicians in forming a therapeutic working alliance with primitive personalities. This is because such individuals lack the capacity for self and object constancy, are unable to sustain a sense of pleasure in relationships, and tend to form pathological symbiotic adaptations in which one party is exploited as the "possession" of the other.

Work with primitive personalities often involves dealing with what is termed *pseudoinsight,* repetitive sequences of apparent insight and understanding, followed by seemingly total forgetting. Interactions which, at the time of their occurrence, may have been viewed as meaningful and relevant seem to vanish from the patient's memory, as if they never took place. This is similar, we may note, to the problems of therapeutic continuity experienced by patients with organic memory disturbances and impaired conceptualization. What accounts for these discouraging cycles in the case of primitive personalities is their characteristic lack of integration, absence of self or object constancy, global destructiveness, and the inability to represent and sustain affective experiences. Again, all these elements are reminiscent of the problems in adaptation experienced by patients with frontal lobe injury.

Many clinicians, including Masterson (1988) and Robbins (1989), have noted the overall refractoriness of primitive personalities to accepting and utilizing interpretations in general. If a patient has no internally experienced emotional referent for the thoughts, feelings, and contradictions that emerge in therapy, he or she may feel misunderstood or criticized, rather than enlightened, by the therapist's interpretive comments—similar to Lewis and Rosenberg's (1990) characterization of psychotherapy as a "burden" to many brain injured patients.

Robbins (1989) proposes a cognitively oriented psychoanalytic technique to treat primitive personalities, the elements of which may sound familiar to those clinicians applying the modalities of brain injury psychotherapy discussed above. Robbins' (1989) technique requires a process of clarification and interpretation directed more toward these patients' unusual cognitive processes and affective deficits than toward their putative unconscious conflicts and defenses. Such cognitively oriented psychodynamic psychotherapy first addresses the question of *how* the patient constructs meaning from his or her experience, and only secondarily explores *what* that meaning might be. Rather than uncovering conflict, the emphasis of psychotherapy with primitive personalities, says Robbins (1989), should be an educative one—we might say a rehabilitative one. For these individuals, analysis of cognition and affect occupies the central position that analysis of conflict and defense occupies in the treatment of other, more integrated patients. Via the therapeutic relationship, the patient's new self is constructed out of the tangible, real-world, neuropsychodynamically adaptive elements of thought, feeling, and action, and thus serves as the scaffolding upon which a new, more integrated personality structure can evolve.

CONCLUSIONS: CONTINUITY, NOT DICHOTOMY

Back to the question of "what we do for" our patients. Perhaps the confusion of some of our colleagues as to the efficacy of the kinds of historical and contemporary therapeutic approaches discussed in this chapter derives from a conceptual misunderstanding of the "purposes" of psychotherapy as a whole.

Guze (1988) discusses two predominant contemporary models of psychotherapy. The first of these, the *etiological* view, is based on the premise that the psychotherapeutic process provides a basis for exposing the complex psychodynamic driving forces responsible for the patient's symptoms and life distress, and that such an approach is, indeed, the only legitimate way of understanding and treating the disorder. Since the success of the treatment depends on the validity of the model, to the extent that the etiological hypotheses are flawed, the justification for the psychotherapy is undermined.

The second approach to psychotherapy described by Guze (1988) is the *rehabilitative* view which approaches the patient's disorder without any obligatory assumptions about etiology, although it may involve careful assessment of the patient's psychological functioning. That is, the patient's symptoms, personality, attitudes, emotions, perceptions, strengths, weaknesses, expectations, and relationships are all evaluated, but without assuming any etiological hypothesis concerning the presenting disorder. The aim is to help the patient understand him- or herself better and, with the aid of the therapist, function more effectively, with less discomfort and less disability, even if there occurs little "insight" as to why the patient's problems began or how the patient's personality developed. A clinical analogy would be to physical therapy, or physical rehabilitation, which is indicated for a wide variety of orthopedic, neurologic, and other syndromes. This form of treatment is nonspecific in that it does not necessarily deal with putative causal conditions or pathogenetic factors. It takes into consideration age, strength, personality, previous skills, etc., in an attempt to foster recovery or improvement in physical disability, but its practitioners need not accept any particular theory of etiology to account for the syndromes they treat.

Undoubtedly, effective psychotherapy combines elements of both the etiological and the rehabilitative approaches, in different proportions for different types of patients and problems (Miller, 1993b). Indeed, many of the psychotherapists whose work has been reviewed here have attempted to tread a path between theoretical coherence and clinical practicality. From the material reviewed in this chapter, we may conclude that what psychotherapy with organic patients and those with "functional" disorders of personality share in common is, first, an emphasis on shoring up the fragile ego structure, the sense of self—indeed, the patient's core identity—before trying to explicate and resolve dynamic–conflictual issues (Miller, 1993a, 1998a, 1998b, in press). In some cases, the self has been shattered by acquired brain injury; in others, it never fully developed due partly to anomalous neurodevelopmental processes which we are only beginning to understand. In both cases, however, it requires our sharpest clinical skills to evaluate and treat these challenging patients, and our efforts must begin with an understanding of our history and a continuing search for unities.

REFERENCES

Begun, J. H. (1976). The sociopathic or psychopathic personality. *International Journal of Social Psychiatry, 14,* 965–975.

Ben-Yishay, Y., & Diller, L. (1983). Cognitive remediation. In E. A. Griffith, M. Bond, & J. Miller (Eds.), *Rehabilitation of the head injured adult* (pp. 367–380). Philadelphia: F. A. Davis.

Ben-Yishay, Y., & Diller, L. (1993). Cognitive remediation in traumatic brain injury: Update and issues. *Archives of Physical Medicine and Rehabilitation, 74,* 204–213.

Carberry, H., & Burd, B. (1985). The use of psychological theory and content as a media in the cognitive and social training of head injured patients. *Cognitive Rehabilitation, 3,* 8–10.

Carberry, H., & Burd, B. (1986). Individual psychotherapy with the brain injured adult. *Cognitive Rehabilitation, 4,* 22–24.

Erickson, R., & Burton, M. (1986). Working with psychiatric patients with cognitive deficits. *Cognitive Rehabilitation, 4,* 26–31.

Freud, S. (1953). The interpretation of dreams. In J. Strachey (Ed.), *The standard edition of the complete psychological works of Sigmund Freud* (Vols. 4 & 5). London: Hogarth Press. (Original work published 1900)

Freud, S. (1957). The unconscious. In J. Strachey (Ed.), *The standard edition of the complete psychological works of Sigmund Freud* (Vol.

14; pp. 159–204). London: Hogarth Press. (Original work published 1915)

Freud, S. (1961). The ego and the id. In J. Strachey (Ed.), *The standard edition of the complete psychological works of Sigmund Freud* (Vol. 19; pp. 1–59). London: Hogarth Press. (Original work published 1923).

Gardner, R. W., Holzman, P. S., Klein, G. S., Linton, H. B., & Spence, D. P. (1959). Cognitive control: A study of individual consistencies in cognitive behavior. *Psychological Issues, 1–* Monogr. 4. New York: International Universities Press.

Goldstein, K. (1952). The effect of brain damage on the personality. *Psychiatry, 15,* 245–260.

Goldstein, K., & Scheerer, M. (1941). Abstract and concrete behavior: An experimental study with special tests. *Psychological Monographs, 43,* 1–151.

Guze, S. B. (1988). Psychotherapy and the etiology of psychiatric disorders. *Psychiatric Developments, 3,* 183–193.

Hartmann, H. (1958). *Ego psychology and the problem of adaptation.* New York: International Universities Press. (Original work published 1939)

Klein, G. S. (1954). Need and regulation. In M. R. Jones (Ed.), *Nebraska symposium on motivation.* Lincoln: University of Nebraska Press.

Klein, G. S. (1958). Cognitive control and motivation. In G. Lindzey (Ed.), *Assessment of human motives.* New York: Rinehart.

Langer, K. G. (1992). Psychotherapy with the neuropsychologically impaired adult. *American Journal of Psychotherapy, 46,* 620–639.

Lewis, L., Allen, J. G., & Frieswyk, S. (1983). The assessment of interacting organic and functional factors in a psychiatric population. *Clinical Neuropsychology, 5,* 65–68.

Lewis, L., & Rosenberg, S. J. (1990). Psychoanalytic psychotherapy with brain-injured adult psychiatric patients. *Journal of Nervous and Mental Disease, 178,* 69–77.

Luria, A. R. (1973). *The working brain: An introduction to neuropsychology.* New York: Basic Books.

Luria, A. R. (1980). *Higher cortical functions in man* (2nd ed.). New York: Basic Books.

Masterson, J. F. (1988). *The search for the real self: Unmasking the personality disorders of our age.* New York: Free Press.

Miller, L. (1990). *Inner natures: Brain, self and personality.* New York: St. Martin's Press.

Miller, L. (1991). *Freud's brain: Neuropsychodynamic foundations of psychoanalysis.* New York: Guilford.

Miller, L. (1993a). *Psychotherapy of the brain-injured patient: Reclaiming the shattered self.* New York: Norton.

Miller, L. (1993b). Who are the best psychotherapists? Qualities of the effective practitioner. *Psychotherapy in Private Practice, 12,* 1–18.

Miller, L. (1997). Freud and consciousness: The first one hundred years of neuropsychodynamics in theory and clinical practice. *Seminars in Neurology, 17,* 171–177.

Miller, L. (1998a). *Shocks to the system: Psychotherapy of traumatic disability syndromes.* New York: Norton.

Miller, L. (1998b). Ego autonomy and the healthy personality: Psychodynamics, cognitive style, and clinical implications. *Psychoanalytic Review, 85,* 423–448.

Miller, L. (in press). Sex differences in personality and psychopathology: Neuropsychology, psychodynamics, and cognitive style. In M. Schulman (Ed.), *Human sexuality: A psychoanalytic perspective.* New York: International Universities Press.

Millon, T. (1981). *Disorders of personality: DSM-III, Axis II.* New York: Wiley.

Millon, T. (1990). *Toward a new personology: An evolutionary model.* New York: Wiley.

Prigatano, G. P. (1991). Disordered mind, wounded soul: The emerging role of psychotherapy in rehabilitation after brain injury. *Journal of Head Trauma Rehabilitation, 6,* 1–10.

Prigatano, G. P., Fordyce, D. J., Zeiner, H. K., Roueche, J. R., Pepping, M., & Wood, B. C. (1986). *Neuropsychological rehabilitation after brain injury.* Baltimore: Johns Hopkins University Press.

Rapaport, D., Gill, M. M., & Schafer, R. (1968). *Diagnostic psychological testing* (rev. ed., Edited by R. R. Holt). New York: International Universities Press.

Robbins, M. (1989). Primitive personality organization as an interpersonally adaptive modification of cognition and affect. *International Journal of Psycho-Analysis, 70,* 443–459.

Shapiro, D. (1965). *Neurotic styles.* New York: Basic Books.

Shapiro, D. (1989). *Psychotherapy of neurotic character.* New York: Basic Books.

Small, L. (1973). *Neuropsychodiagnosis in psychotherapy.* New York: Brunner/Mazel.

Small, L. (1980). *Neuropsychodiagnosis in psychotherapy* (rev. ed.). New York: Brunner/Mazel.

3.

Ethical Challenges

Robert M. Gordon, Psy.D.

Ethics are the values, principles, and norms assumed in a given cultural or professional setting and are utilized in determining appropriate conduct. While literature in the field of bioethics has proliferated, examples and models discussed therein predominantly address emergency or acute medical care rather than rehabilitation medical settings (Caplan, Callahan, & Haas, 1987).

Acute care and rehabilitation medicine can be viewed as two endpoints on a continuum of goals within health care. The primary objective of acute medical care is immediate cure, while the goals of rehabilitation are improvement in overall functioning over an extended period of time. Rehabilitation rarely involves the dramatic cure or the life-saving technology found in acute care settings. Consequently, the moral and ethical questions arising in rehabilitation tend to be different from existing ethical models addressing issues of acute care (Caplan et al., 1987).

In medical rehabilitation, professionals are more likely to confront conditions that are chronic, irreversible, and relatively stable (Caplan et al., 1987). Jennings (1993) described the overall goal of rehabilitation as the revitalization of the patient's power to live a meaningful life. Rehabilitation professionals attempt to reduce the impact of disability by enhancing compensatory functional abilities through skills retraining and environmental modification (Haas, 1987). Through rehabilitation, patients are encouraged to strive toward the highest levels of autonomy possible given the limitations and obstacles imposed by the disability (Purtillo, 1988).

MODELS OF ETHICAL DECISION MAKING

Three ethical models of physician–patient decision making dominate the field of medicine. These include the traditional model of medical paternalism, as well as the contractual and the educational models (Caplan et al., 1987). These models parallel what Siegler (1993) described as the three phases of medicine—the age of the doctor, the age of the patient, and the age of the payer.

A fourth model particularly relevant to rehabilitation medicine, the relational perspectivistic model, best represents the psychological challenges and ethical complexities of working with patients experiencing neurological impairment. This model, which has not been applied to medical ethical decision making, will be discussed at length later in this chapter.

The Traditional Model: Medical Paternalism

The "Age of the Doctor" characterized medical care from about 500 BCE to around 1965 (Siegler, 1993). In this model, decisions are based principally on the physician's ability to prognosticate about the patient. Paternalism was the caregiver's method of relating to patients. The physician believed that he or she was entitled to act in the presumed best interest of a patient without his or her consent. The paternalistic model depicted the physician, given his or her specialized knowledge, as an active patient advocate (Caplan et al., 1987). Historically, many physicians in the United States and other Western nations did not perceive the patients' best interest to involve informing them of the diagnosis or prognosis. As recently as the 1950s, physicians typically withheld information from seriously or terminally ill patients. They rationalized withholding bad news on the grounds that it would be harmful or that patients preferred not to know negative truths (Caplan, 1988).

Contractual Model

Critics of the paternalistic model agreed that patients had minimal autonomy in contesting physicians' recommendations. These critics advocated for more egalitarian physician–patient relationships and decision making (Caplan et al., 1987). By 1965, the spectrum of medical interventions began to change rapidly with advances in kidney dialysis, transplantation surgeries, chemotherapies and intensive care medicine. During this phase of medicine involving complex choices regarding care, patients and their families increasingly challenged the absolute power of the physician and requested greater participation in the decision-making process. The principles of informed consent and confidentiality thus became more prominent (Siegler, 1993).

The opponents of medical paternalism advocated a more democratic model of the physician–patient relationship based on contract theory and reflecting the rapid social changes of the 1960s. The doctrine of the patient's informed consent was a central feature of this model. The contractual model assumed that the patient was competent to make rational choices and was motivated to do so. From this perspective, physicians should provide optimal medical care, but only that desired and accepted by the patient. Patients had the right to refuse potentially beneficial care if their decisions were based on voluntary informed choice (Caplan et al., 1987). As this model increasingly became a central component of all medical and ethical decision making, a parallel shift in focus occurred in clinical practice involving the increased sharing of information regarding diagnosis and prognosis (Caplan et al., 1987).

The Educational Model

The educational model emphasizes a flexible use of paternalistic and educational interventions depending on the phase of rehabilitation. During the initial phases of rehabilitation, patients with neurological impairments commonly experience considerable distress, anxiety, and disorientation, rendering rational choices difficult. Caplan (1988) has advocated that physicians and other health care professionals be allowed more latitude during this initial phase of treatment than the contractual model provides. The caregiver's role in the educational model could be paternalistic in the service of eventually restoring or enhancing the neurologically impaired patient's long-term autonomy. In fact, patients psychologically capable of making treatment decisions need time to adjust to new illnesses or disabilities, as well as to process the information they are given. In the view of Caplan et al. (1987), the onset of an unexpected neurological impairment warrants great sensitivity by health care providers regarding the patient's readiness to hear and retain important information. The educational model also requires, however, that the rehabilitation team strive to restore patient autonomy as quickly as possible by providing detailed information regarding the course of treatment and risks and benefits of alternative approaches, as well as involving the patient and family actively in goal-setting.

The Relational–Perspectivistic Model

An alternative approach to physician–patient interaction and ethical decision making is based on the relational–perspectivistic model described in the recent psychoanalytic literature (Aron, 1996). This paradigm of ethical decision making considers the importance of the following components: (1) values;

(2) patients' and their families' transference reactions; (3) staff countertransference feelings; (4) institutional, social, and cultural context (including the impact of insurance and managed care companies); and (5) the importance of ongoing negotiation.

This model takes into consideration a new development in medical care: the impact of financial and insurance concerns on the patient and health care providers in the current "Age of the Payer" (Siegler, 1993), and it runs parallel with the third phase of medicine—the age of the payer (Siegler, 1993). The national attempt to control escalating costs, which emerged in 1983 when the concept of diagnostic related groups (DRGs) came into being, metamorphized the traditional dyadic physician–patient relationship to a triadic relationship, with considerable power and influence over all aspects of decision making being held by managed care organizations (Kirschner, 1995).

The relational–perspectivistic model is strongly influenced by Hoffman's writings on social constructivism (1991, 1992). This paradigm emphasizes the critical role of the observer in shaping, constructing, and organizing the patient's reality. This constructivistic perspective maintains that "objective reality" varies considerably among different cultures (Malec, 1993). Thus, the relational–perspectivistic approach stresses the ambiguity of reality: Each individual involved in making ethical decisions has his or her plausible view of the situation. Knowledge is perspectival and other beliefs, value systems, and centers of subjectivity are acknowledged (Aron, 1996). This does not imply that every construction of the patient's experience is equally valid or accurate. The patient's experience, despite its highly ambiguous nature, consists of particular constraints of interpretation analogous to form level on the Rorschach (Mitchell, 1997). By highlighting the importance of meaning and values, ethical decisions are arrived at through an ongoing dialogue between the patient, family, and interdisciplinary staff.

Understanding the critical role that values play in the relational perspective sheds light on this fourth model of decision making. Impairments in speech, ambulation, perception, reading, memory, and activities of daily living have different meanings for different patients, family members, and health care providers (Caplan et al., 1987). Patients entering a rehabilitation setting encounter a novel situation with differing expectations and demands reflecting underlying values (Wegener, 1996). Rehabilitation settings promote values such as independence, maximum effort without complaining, and accepting pain at the expense of comfort and nurturance (Wegener, 1996). Gunther (1987) stated that there is a strong emphasis in rehabilitation settings on performance-oriented goal attainment. The complexity of quality of life concerns tend to be minimized as focus is placed on treatment outcomes, efficiency, accountability, and compliance (Wegener, 1996). Holmes (1996) believed that values tend to have a powerful unconscious influence on attitudes and behaviors. Consciously held values, however, may be defensive efforts to minimize the impact of unconscious feelings of hatred, envy, guilt and frustration. Holmes advocated that therapists carefully explore and monitor how their values affect their work, a process described as gaining awareness of ethical countertransference.

Transference and countertransference reactions are also critical features of the relational–perspectivistic model. Transference and countertransference define the global, interactive experience of the patient and the therapist. Each is assumed to respond to the real participation of the other, shaped by internal conflicts, character, values, and past experiences. Neither transference nor countertransference are assumed to be distortions. The patient's transference reactions are patterned attempts by the patient to relate to others, protect the self, and regulate levels of closeness and privacy. Conversely, the therapist's countertransference is an effort to relate to the patient, protect the self, and regulate his or her level of intimacy or distance from the patient (Gordon with Aron, Mitchell, & Davies, 1998). Transference and countertransference reactions are extremely common events and should be examined as actions within a specific context, with specific aims (Mitchell, 1997). In addition, both the therapist and patient are seen as the initiators of transference–countertransference conflicts and impasses (Aron, 1996).

From a relational perspectivistic model, transference and countertransference are mutual creations by patient and analyst. Patients evoke specific feelings, thoughts, and memories in the therapist, while the therapist's own defenses, coping styles, values, and unconscious motivations ultimately determine the countertransference response (Gabbard, 1995). Transference can be described as a selectivity in awareness or rigidity in perception (Fiscalini, 1995). Hoffman (1983) believed that transference operates like a "Geiger counter," with past experiences causing patients to selectively perceive meaning in situations or notice qualities and motivations in others that might be insignificant to someone else.

Psychologists working with adults who are neurologically impaired are confronted with intensive and ongoing patient transferences, events that are increased by several factors in a rehabilitation setting: the traumatic and sudden disorganization of the adult patient's personality structure and defensive system, the inevitable psychological regression, and the prolonged state of physical dependency (Gunther, 1987). Prominent countertransference reactions in staff members include rage and hatred toward patients who may consistently frustrate their best therapeutic efforts, as well as the caregiver's own feelings of helplessness, hopelessness, and fears of their own mortality and limitations (Gans, 1983; Gunther, 1987).

ETHICAL CHALLENGES IN PSYCHOTHERAPY WITH BRAIN-INJURED ADULTS

The major ethical challenges in psychotherapy with adults experiencing a neurological impairment encompass clinical dilemmas regarding: (1) decision making; (2) refusal of treatment; (3) potential dangerousness; (4) patient and staff conflict; and (5) broader philosophical issues regarding the overall goals of rehabilitation (Jennings, 1993). This population particularly challenges the therapist's ideals of autonomy, self-determination, and independence (Jennings, 1993).

Ethical considerations must shape the therapist's approach to the obstacles and daily realities confronting individuals adjusting to neurological impairment. Unrealistic notions of ideal autonomy may lead the patient to experience disappointment and conflict, rather than empowerment and self-respect. Concrete and contextual descriptions of potential independence are needed to deal with the patient's daily concerns after experiencing a sudden and unexpected neurological impairment.

Three ethical issues provide the foundation for any potential psychotherapeutic encounter: quality of life, the nature of autonomy, and decision making. The complexity and depth of ethical challenges in psychotherapy are demonstrated by carefully exploring these concepts.

Quality of Life

Quality of life is a multidimensional and interactive concept that consists of the overall level of personal satisfaction with objective life conditions such as physical, material, social, and emotional well-being (Felce & Perry, 1996). Values such as self-determination, autonomy, and personal choice are critical components in determining life satisfaction (Hughes & Hwang, 1996). An individual's subjective sense of well-being is highly related to that which is most meaningful in life (Dresser & Whitehouse, 1994). One of the central features of our democratic society is a respect for pluralism. We expect and encourage individuals to express diverse perspectives of the meaning and ultimate purpose of human life. Pluralism posits that no one standard exists measuring "good" for a patient experiencing a neurological impairment. Psychotherapeutic interventions and decision making depend on highly specific conceptions of the meaning of human life (Emanuel, 1987).

Common emotional themes for individuals experiencing a neurological impairment include: (1) loss of a sense of self-cohesion and integrity; (2) feelings of helplessness and vulnerability; (3) fears of an uncertain future; and (4) existential issues of loss of control over events and one's mortality (Langer, 1992). These themes all relate to the patient's and caregiver's conception of what constitutes a qualitatively meaningful life.

Emanuel (1987) described five perspectives on a purposeful existence for patients who are experiencing significant neurological impairment: (1) vitalism; (2) hedonism; (3) interpersonal orientation; (4) autonomous emphasis; and (5) utilitarianism. The physical or vitalism view advocates that life alone, whatever the degree of suffering, is meaningful and purposeful. A consequence of this perspective is that any intervention that maintains or improves physical existence, regardless of issues of pain, is beneficial to the patient. In contrast, the hedonistic perspective stresses that pleasure, and the avoidance of significant pain and suffering, is the most critical component in defining an acceptable life. The interpersonal orientation highlights the meaning and satisfaction derived from the love and care of interpersonal relationships. The autonomy paradigm, on the other hand, stresses the importance of self-determination and freedom from the coercive control of others. In this view, when an individual is not capable of making intentional and informed decisions (Romano, 1989), medical interventions cease to be useful. The fifth, or utilitarian, perspective stresses the collective total of pain and pleasure experienced by all individuals involved in the decision process as the ultimate criteria of determining "an acceptable existence." Medical interventions are beneficial only if collective pleasure is greater than the pain experienced by the entire family system (Emanuel, 1987). These five perspectives justify different types and intensities of treatment, and can be considered components of the therapist's ethical countertransference (Holmes, 1996). Different diagnoses, issues in treatment, and the patients' personality traits and family dynamics may evoke varying ethical countertransference reactions in the therapist.

Autonomy

A frequently unexamined and unconscious aspect of the therapist's ethical countertransference system involves different perspectives on the patient's autonomy. As described in the democratic tradition, the ideal of autonomy depicts the individual as possessing a maximum of independent action and thought, self-determination, and ability to identify desires and interests (Agich, 1990). While this definition is useful in political and legal discussions, it does not fully address the pressing real-life issues arising during psychotherapy with adults experiencing brain injury. A more concrete and contextual definition is needed (Agich, 1990).

Autonomous choices need to be consistent with one's values, beliefs, and life plans. The concept implies that choices, even those that consist of depending on others for physical and emotional care, are reflective of one's basic character. From a relational–perspectivistic viewpoint, autonomy results from contextually situated options that are personally meaningful for those involved (Agich, 1990; Childress, 1990). The choices offered to an individual experiencing a neurological impairment must be personally meaningful, worth making, and reflective of one's unique personality (Agich, 1990), while at the same time taking into consideration the realities posed by the neurological deficit.

A more clinically relevant description of patient autonomy in this context must recognize the influence of professionals and the power of managed care companies and institutional politics and values. This perspective advocates an increased awareness of these underlying forces. Autonomy is not something that precedes interactions with patients and families, but is "an emergent property of the interactive process, not something that can be sheltered from influence, but something that grows through influence" (Mitchell, 1997, p. 21). The caregiver's most constructive protection of patient autonomy is accomplished by acknowledging the interactive and perspectivistic nature of the rehabilitation process (Mitchell, 1997).

Ethical Decision Making

Competency involves the capacity to make decisions for which the individual is accountable and responsible. Individuals need to adequately appreciate the long-term positive and negative implications of decisions, rather than focus exclusively on short-term factual aspects of decisions (Elliott, 1997). Freedman, Stuss, & Gordon (1991) stated that decision-making capacity depends on an ability to retain, process, and understand information, develop and analyze alternative plans, as well as an ability to communicate one's choices. Thus, competency is not a unitary concept. The reality of multiple competencies means that a central question is the patient's ability to perform a specific skill in a particular context (Marson, Schmitt, Ingram, & Harrell, 1994). Professionals' judgments regarding the patient's competency to make decisions should be based on the highest observed level of performance under optimal conditions (Haffey, 1989).

Ethical decision making is complicated by common personality changes that may result from neurological impairment, including poor social judgment and impulsivity, egocentricity, emotional lability, and disinhibition. Typical reactive emotional problems include increased anxiety, depression, irritability, withdrawal, and mistrust of others (Cicerone, 1989). Neurological impairment tends to exacerbate preexisting personality traits and to interfere with coping strategies. These regressions are attributable to a decrease in problem-solving abilities and cognitive flexibility and the stress and anxiety of living with a disability (Langer, 1992).

Among the most ethically challenging tasks in psychotherapy with brain injured adults is decision making. This covers a wide spectrum of dilemmas including managing finances, consenting to medical treatment, giving power of attorney, making a will, choosing a place to live, resuming a job, driving a car, managing a medication schedule, and choosing a level of caregiver assistance (Freedman et al., 1991; Gass & Brown, 1992).

When a psychologist must determine a patient's competence to make decisions, he or she will need to evaluate four different dimensions: (1) the risk–benefit ratio of the decision; (2) patient neuropsychological functioning; (3) patient emotional and motivational factors; and (4) patient understanding of the specific decision that needs to be made.

Consent to Medical Interventions

When dealing with decision-making choices in psychotherapy, the psychologist needs to consider such factors as the risk–benefit ratio (i.e., how much do the potential benefits of the decision outweigh the possible risks?). A lower level of reasoning and understanding is required when a patient gives informed consent to a medical intervention with a beneficial risk–benefit ratio or refuses a treatment with an uncertain chance of success. On the other hand, a higher degree of reasoning and understanding is needed when a patient refuses a medical intervention with a highly beneficial risk–benefit ratio or if the decision poses a significant medical threat to the person (Roth, Meisel, & Lidz, 1977).

When evaluating a neurologically impaired individual's level of competence to consent to medical interventions or other major decisions, a number of neuropsychological variables need to be considered including attentional, memory, language, visuospatial and executive skills, as well as emotional functioning. Alexander (1988, cited in Callahan & Hagglund, 1995) cites a number of risk factors and test scores that can be utilized in making competency determinations, including patient's ability to state fewer than five digits forward, decrease in mental control when performing serial subtraction, inability to encode and recall a list of four words, disorientation, concrete, tangential, or autistic thinking and the presence of such conditions as receptive aprosodia and anosognosia.

Motivational and emotional factors may significantly impact an individual's ability to make responsible decisions (Callahan & Hagglund, 1995). Severe depression will impact the neurologically impaired individual's ability to care about medical decisions, to appreciate the long-term consequences of the decision, and to carefully consider the risks and benefits of the decision (Elliott, 1997). Many studies have found that severely depressed patients have cognitive deficits in reasoning and information processing (Appelbaum, 1997).

A fourth component in evaluating competency to consent to medical interventions involves the patient's understanding of specific aspects of the actual intervention. Venesy (1994) described a number of questions that can be explored in psychotherapy with a neurologically impaired adult faced with a difficult decision regarding a specific medical intervention. The patient should confront his or her level of awareness of medical needs, the imminence of the decision, the patient and his or her physicians' thoughts on the implications of accepting or rejecting treatment, alternative interventions, and the potential benefits and limitations of each choice. Venesy (1994) observed that since competence for decision making may vary among patients, two or three assessments are often necessary.

Moreover, the manner in which treatment choices are presented can have a significant impact on assessment of competency (Callahan & Hagglund, 1995). The patient's level of understanding and recall of information can be affected by the mode of presentation (i.e., visual, auditory), rate of presentation, open-ended versus forced or multiple choice, linguistic or conceptual complexity, degree of extraneous stimulation in the environment, and time of day (Haffey, 1989).

Refusal of Treatment

Refusal of treatment is a multidetermined behavior and has different meanings for each patient as the treatment evolves. Reidy, Crozier, Caplan, Kutys, and Sinnott (1992) used a consultative model to describe a number of steps a psychologist can employ when a patient refuses to participate in aspects of the rehabilitation process. Using strategies from both a behavioral and psychodynamic orientation, the specificity of the refusal should be explored, particularly with respect to whether the refusal is ongoing, sporadic, or acute in nature. The antecedents and the consequences of the behavior should be considered as well as the underlying causes and stated reasons for the refusal. In addition, the patient's significant others should be consulted on whether the reasons for the refusal are consistent with the patient's premorbid character and values. These detailed areas of inquiry will often resolve the dilemma.

Another potential reason for refusal of treatment is projective identification, or an unconscious attempt on the part of

the patient to communicate intense feelings. Projective identification differs from pure projection in that it not only expels
uncomfortable aspects of the self, but also induces the object
of the projection to experience the projection. Individuals who
engage in projective identification are reluctant to experience
or notice within themselves qualities and traits that are recognized critically in others (Mitchell, 1997). Ogden (1979) trans-
formed the concept into an interpersonal construct by
describing projective identification as a process in which a
group of fantasies and accompanying self representations are
deposited into the therapist and are later returned in a modified and less threatening version. The patient unconsciously
attempts to induce in the therapist a particular role or feeling
in order to protect against overwhelming anxiety (Knapp,
1989). Often, refusals of treatment are simply the patient's attempt at communicating feelings of helplessness, fear, and
rage. The positive aspects of projective identification, including
its adaptive function as a form of communicating feelings that
cannot be put into words, needs to be balanced with its disruptive aspects. Refusal of treatment can also be viewed as an attempt at assertiveness and control, or a sign of ineffective
communication patterns between patient and staff.

Venesy (1994) also noted that a patient's refusal of treatment may be affected by the fear and intense anxiety evoked
by the potential intervention stimulated by unconscious associations concerning loss of control, issues involving body integrity, fear of total dependency, and mortality. Other factors that
need to be considered are the accuracy and comprehensiveness
of the information presented to the patient, the consistency or
fluctuation in the patient's mental status and level of orientation, metabolic status, level and tolerance of pain, and the impact of various medications (Venesy, 1994). A case example
will be used to illustrate these concepts.

Case Example 1

Mrs. L, a 68-year-old retiree with a left cerebrovascular accident,
mild expressive aphasia, short-term memory deficits, and a premorbid history of anorexia, refused to participate in any of

her inpatient therapies. She felt that certain members of the treatment team hated her and treated her unjustly. After attending her therapies for the first 2 weeks of her hospitalization, she abruptly refused treatment and subsequently lost a significant amount of weight. The entire rehabilitation team became highly anxious and preoccupied with the case. Mrs. L played staff members against one another. Her primary physician tried to avoid her frequent and frantic pleas for constant and undivided attention. This situation escalated over a 2-week period, and a series of team meetings were held. Staff members contributed to this difficult situation in part by providing inconsistent information regarding her diagnosis and treatment goals. In addition, the patient and her family had an idealized view of the physician. Failing to meet their unrealistically inflated expectations, the physician became the target of unconscious feelings of rage and disappointment (i.e., projective identification). The physician experienced his own hateful reactions, but felt guilty and responded in an overprotective, but unassertive manner. At the team meeting, the physician was given permission to experience his hateful feelings, which were shared by a number of members of the treatment team.

Other members of the interdisciplinary team were more positively disposed toward Mrs. L. They perceived that, underneath a demanding, aggressive facade, she was, in fact, quite needy and attention-seeking. The psychologist, acting as a consultant, maintained that each staff member was playing out a different aspect of Mrs. L's personality and that the patient was inducing the staff to experience her unmanageable feelings. The staff subsequently agreed to refer all questions concerning her diagnosis and treatment program to the physician. It was also decided that an alternative rehabilitation program focusing on her anorexia would be more suitable at the present time.

This case illustrates the difficulties in distinguishing neuropsychological symptoms from premorbid psychiatric problems. The staff increased its awareness of the powerful unconscious forces that impact on their daily work by considering psychoanalytic concepts such as countertransference and projective identification at the team meeting. As Mitchell (1997) has stated, "Projective identification is one way to think about the unconscious processes through which the conflictual richness of experience, too varied to be containable in one mind at any time, becomes distributed in dyads and groups'' (pp. 264–265).

Case Example 2

Mr. R, a 50-year-old male accountant, suffered a right cerebrovascular accident. During a 2-month inpatient rehabilitation process, he had no contact with his accounting firm. A comprehensive neuropsychological evaluation indicated significant deficits in visuomotor planning and inattention to small visual details. Mr. R adamantly stated that all information regarding his medical condition remain confidential since he intended to return to work upon discharge from the hospital. The psychologist was quite concerned about Mr. R's ability to successfully perform his job, given the necessity for close attention to detail and the potentially serious ramifications in the case of errors. Mr. R threatened to sue the psychologist if the medical condition was revealed to business partners. After consulting with his own supervisor, the psychologist scheduled a meeting with Mr. R, his wife, and physician to focus on the risks and benefits inherent in resuming full-time employment. Daily problems that Mr. R had noted and expressed during his psychotherapy sessions, as well as the confirmation of these problems disclosed in neuropsychological testing, were discussed. Mr. R and his wife expressed their fears regarding finances, the threatened loss of role identities, and the impact of these changes. A compromise was reached, and Mr. R agreed to attend cognitive remediation for a 4-month period and subsequently worked on a part-time basis under close supervision. Mr. R was able to share some of his deficits with his partners, who responded in a flexible and supportive manner.

This case highlights the need to protect the patient and potential third parties. By involving significant others at the team meeting, a helpful transition phase was made feasible. Alerting Mr. R's firm was viewed as a last resort. Even then, it would have occurred only with the approval of the patient and his wife in order to safeguard confidentiality and the patient's sense of integrity. If Mr. R had been in a position in which the health of others was in danger (i.e., a surgeon), then the need to protect third parties would have been considered even more rigorously.

Dangerousness

The clinical challenges posed by an adult who is neurologically impaired who decides to resume driving involve ethical issues concerning caregiver's duty to protect third parties and patient confidentiality. The Tarasoff ruling of a mandated duty to protect has been extended to unspecified victims of impaired drivers and their physicians (Brittain, Frances, & Barth, 1995). If a patient who is neurologically impaired injures another person while driving, the victim can sue the physician working with the patient. The victim must prove, however, that the physician knew that the patient was driving, failed to notify law enforcement or licensing authorities (i.e., Department of Motor Vehicles), did not confront the patient or the patient's legal representative about the fact that driving was dangerous and forbidden, and that the harm to the victim was a direct consequence of a foreseeable cognitive mistake by the patient (Beresford, 1996).

Case Example 3

Mr. S, 48 years old, suffered a traumatic brain injury as a result of a motor vehicle accident. Computed tomography (CT) of the brain revealed bilateral frontal hematomas. During his inpatient hospitalization course, Mr. S exhibited poor judgment, impulsivity, and a general lack of awareness of his deficits and the implications of these problems on activities of daily living. A serious ethical dilemma arose when Mr. S told the psychologist during a session that he wished to resume driving upon his discharge. Mr. S became enraged when the psychologist expressed her concerns over his stated intention. Feedback from neuropsychological testing and discussions with his occupational therapist regarding his impulsivity and poor planning skills had minimal impact, except to increase his sense of rigidity and determination to drive.

A team meeting was held with Mr. S's wife, eldest son, psychologist, occupational therapist, and physician. At this meeting, Mr. S was able to express his rage over his lack of independence and his perception of his family's overprotective and infantilizing response to his disability. The psychologist posed the question to the patient and family as to how they would feel if the patient's grandson was seriously injured by an impaired driver. This question and the emotionally cathartic discussion resulted in a mutual decision by the entire family to have a comprehensive driver evaluation.

The ethical obligation to protect neurologically impaired adults and potential victims does not imply that all those with neurological injuries are dangerous drivers. Some patients with more focal lesions are capable drivers. The assessment of driving capacity needs to be carefully evaluated on an ongoing basis by a specialist.

Conflicts Between Patients, Families, and Staff

Among the most complex and anxiety-provoking challenges confronting health care professionals are the conflicts between patients, their families, and the treatment team on treatment and financial decisions. These conflicts often involve issues of hope, denial, and awareness. Family members may perceive denial as the other face of hope, and there may be some benefits derived from this "optimism," but professionals may, with good reason, experience the denial as the other face of disaster.

Hope is comprised of both cognitive and affective components. When hope is experienced as an expectation regarding the high attainability of a goal or anticipated future, its cognitive aspect is emphasized (Buechler, 1995). Buechler differentiated a passive longing for a more satisfying future, which consists of the wishful expectation that a person, event, spiritual faith or time itself, will bring fulfillment and healing and hope as an active affect. As an active motivating force, change occurs as a result of effort and taking personal responsibility. Hope can be understood only in the context of other emotions such as joy, curiosity, dread, and fear (Mitchell, 1993; Buechler, 1995).

Hope is a concept that crystallizes when contrasted with denial, awareness, and dissociation. Langer and Padrone (1992) proposed a tripartite model of understanding and working clinically with denial and awareness. The individual may: (1) lack the required information regarding their own neurological condition; (2) have the necessary factual information about their condition, but minimize the implication of this knowledge; or (3) utilize the coping strategy of denial. In this frequently encountered and normal reaction to trauma, the individual possesses the knowledge and has the cognitive and emotional capacity to comprehend the implication of this information, but behaves in a manner that indicates a belief that the information is not accurate. The individual perceives the information as too painful and anxiety provoking.

Langer and Padrone (1992) stated that, in the beginning phase of acute rehabilitation, incomplete awareness of deficits is frequently observed because patients have not had the opportunity to discover their limitations on their own. With the gradual and difficult process of attempting activities of daily living, memory, visuospatial and attentional, gross and fine motor tasks in the hospital and at home, the adult with brain injury is more likely to gain awareness of his or her own problems. In some cases, patients should be permitted to maintain some degree of denial if it does not significantly interfere with their rehabilitation and daily functioning. Denial is an appropriate and adaptive coping strategy in the earlier stages of adjustment to brain injury. It provides a transitional period of time to adapt to an overwhelming situation.

The defensive use of denial, however, needs to be differentiated from dissociation. According to Bromberg (1994) and Davies (1996), trauma creates affects and thoughts that cannot be integrated by the individual. Bromberg stated that dissociation is a protection against overwhelming anxiety that can result in self-fragmentation. The individual's inability to reflect on experience occurs out of necessity (Stern, 1997). Stern (1997) contrasted dissociation in response to trauma with expectable dissociation, which he delineates as an unconscious decision not to interpret and linguistically encode experience. To dissociate means to constrict the range and depth of interpretations one makes of experience. Bromberg (1994), Davies and Frawley (1994), and Stern (1996) emphasized that dissociated self-states cannot be put directly into words and can be discovered only through the impact on the patient–therapist interaction.

Case Example 4

Mr. H, 21 years old, was admitted to an inpatient rehabilitation program with a mild traumatic brain injury and a fractured ankle and femur. Mr. H was the driver of a car in which his older brother died. Mr. H came from a strong patriarchal family that promoted values such as perseverance, stoicism, and achievement. During the initial phase of rehabilitation, Mr. H was highly anxious and disoriented as to time and place. He had dissociated the accident and was experiencing nightmares. During the second week of hospitalization, Mr. H's ability to focus and his level of orientation improved. A neuropsychological evaluation was conducted at this time. Mr. H was quite concerned with his performance and frequently asked for immediate feedback. He had extremely high expectations for himself, which was also an important feature of his premorbid personality. His neuropsychological deficits included reduced information processing speed, and difficulties with complex attentional tasks and visuomotor skills when timed.

A number of staff and family conflicts emerged during the second week of rehabilitation. Mr. H's father attended all his physical, occupational, and speech therapy sessions, and wanted to be present during the neuropsychological evaluation. He firmly stated that he did not want his son to be told that his older brother died in the accident, believing that this knowledge would significantly interfere with his surviving son's ability to remain strong and focused. During physical therapy sessions, Mr. H's father commanded and pressured his son to work harder and faster. It appeared that Mr. H's family held the unconscious fantasy that, if Mr. H worked hard and fast enough, his complete recovery would miraculously bring back his deceased brother. Mr. H's father's constant and manic presence provoked a high degree of anxiety in the staff, who felt that Mr. H needed more time and independence to discover his own limitations and mourn his losses. The father denied that there were any changes in Mr. H's status except for his broken leg and ankle. While Mr. H had some awareness of changes in his neurological status, he tended to minimize the implications or severity. He also used humor and externalized blame as primary defenses. Mr. H and his parents believed that he could return to college on a full-time basis upon his discharge.

The staff became quite concerned over the father's intrusive involvement and desire to keep his son from learning about his brother's death. A family meeting was held with Mr. H's physician, psychologist, social worker, and physical and occupational therapist. Mr. H's father's goals appeared to be a combination of denial of his son's limitations and an unrealistic hope that more activity and effort would lead to a complete cure. The staff strongly recommended that Mr. H be told of his brother's death because he was beginning to ask questions about his brother. They expressed concern about how Mr. H would react if he accidentally found out. The psychologist supported the father's values of perseverance and achievement and his dedication to his son's rehabilitation. In addition, the father's hopeful feelings were validated, but it was recommended that a more patient and gradual attitude toward his son's progress be taken. Staff also recommended that the father not attend therapy sessions due to his son's growing anxiety and self-criticism if he failed to reach goals immediately. Bereavement counseling for the family as well as Mr. H's return to college on a part-time basis were suggested.

Mr. H's father agreed not to attend his son's therapy session, but refused the suggestion of family counseling or his son's returning to college on a part-time basis. He did agree, after considerable discussion, that the psychologist could contact Mr. H's college advisor regarding ancillary interventions that would increase his chances of succeeding at school. The psychologist informed the advisor of specific remediation strategies that would increase the student's chances of success. Therefore, someone at the school needed to take an active role in providing these interventions.

This case illustrates the complex family and staff conflicts that emerge when issues of hope, denial, dissociation, and individual and family personality traits and values collide. Clinical interventions to handle denial and unrealistic hope should be carefully considered at team meetings. In this case, staff felt that the withholding of information about Mr. H's brother and his father's constant pressure interfered with Mr. H's rehabilitation and emotional functioning, while returning to school on a full-time basis posed a lower degree of risk.

Case Example 5

Mr. C, 55 years old, sustained a moderate traumatic brain injury as a result of a motor vehicle accident. He was observed spending and giving away money at an alarming rate. The large financial settlement that he had been awarded had dwindled to half its original amount. Mr. C's wife and two children became extremely distressed when they were notified by Mr. C that he had revised his will and was leaving most of his money to his closest friend and younger brother. Both had visited Mr. C on a regular basis during his extended inpatient rehabilitation program. Mr. C's wife and children became outraged and decided to take legal steps to declare Mr. C incompetent. Mr. C became highly anxious about this possibility. He agreed to attend an outpatient brain injury program where he completed an extensive neuropsychological evaluation.

The results of the testing indicated that Mr. C had significant left frontal and temporal impairment, including short-term auditory memory deficits, and difficulty shifting sets and evaluating the effectiveness of problem-solving strategies. Although Mr. C was able to perform simple calculations and use a calculator, he was unable to balance a checkbook and to budget a monthly expense task. He was able, however, to express his disappointment and hurt feelings toward his wife and children. He felt they were not sufficiently involved during his rehabilitation program and generally showed an apathetic attitude toward him and his neurological condition. He was also able to state the reasons why he wanted to leave his money to his closest friend and brother. The case eventually went to court and the judge ruled that Mr. C's brother would be appointed guardian of his financial affairs. The judge also decided that Mr. C's revised will was valid because Mr. C was able to reliably express whom he was leaving the money to and the reasons for this decision.

This case describes the complexities of differentiating legal and neuropsychological aspects of competency. Cognitive impairment may cause inattention to financial responsibilities, managing bank accounts, and impulsive spending, which can have a significant impact on the family (Beresford, 1996). Current legal decisions usually restrict a guardian's powers to those areas affected by the individual's limitations and allow for autonomous functioning in areas that are likely to pose minimal risk (Beresford, 1996). In this case, Mr. C's reckless and impulsive spending was found to pose a greater threat to his own and to his family's security than his decision to revise his will. In addition, his decision to revise his will could be explored in greater detail during individual and family therapy sessions during the upcoming years and could be considered a reversible decision.

CONCLUDING REMARKS

The use of a relational–perspectivistic model of ethical decision making provides a rich foundation of practical concepts such as quality of life, autonomy, hope, projective identification, ethical countertransference, and the importance of meaning and context. These philosophical principles and psychoanalytic ideas add depth and complexity to discussions of ethical dilemmas regarding adults with neurological impairment. It provides a framework that is most consistent with the difficult, day-to-day challenges posed in psychotherapy and rehabilitation. This model stresses that autonomy and quality of life are achievements that are mutually discovered and created by the patient, family, and health care professional. These goals are not concepts that are applied identically to each patient, but are unique accomplishments that are consistent with the individual patient's character, values, and culture.

In order to arrive at optimal ethical decisions in rehabilitation, it is advisable to organize family and team meetings at which all parties can express their different perspectives and concerns, and where each member of the rehabilitation team and each family member may contribute their unique viewpoints. The process of ethical decision making provides an opportunity to learn other disciplines' perspectives. Ultimately, the most significant teacher may well be the patient.

REFERENCES

Agich, G. (1990). Reassessing autonomy in long-term care. *Hastings Center Report, 20*, 12–17.

Alexander, M. (1988). Clinical determination of mental competence: A theoretical and a retrospective study. *Archives of Neurology, 45*, 23–26.

Appelbaum, P. S. (1997). Rethinking the conduct of psychiatric research. *Archives of General Psychiatry, 54*, 117–120.

Aron, L. (1996). *A meeting of minds: Mutuality in psychoanalysis.* Hillsdale, NJ: Analytic Press.

Beresford, H. R. (1996). The determination of competency in the brain-injured person. In R. W. Evans (Ed.), *Neurology and trauma* (pp. 626–633). Philadelphia, PA: W. B. Saunders.

Brittain, J. L., Frances, J. P., & Barth, J. T. (1995). Ethical issues in neuropsychological practice reported by ABCN diplomats. *Advances in Medical Psychotherapy, 8*, 1–22.

Bromberg, P. (1994). "Speak! That I may see you": Some reflections on dissociation, reality and psychoanalytic listening. *Psychoanalytic Dialogues, 4*, 517–548.

Buechler, S. (1995). Hope as inspiration in psychoanalysis. *Psychoanalytic Dialogues, 5*, 63–74.

Callahan, C. D., & Hagglund, K. J. (1995). Comparing neuropsychological and psychiatric evaluations of competency in rehabilitation: A case example. *Archives of Physical Medicine and Rehabilitation, 76,* 909–912.

Caplan, A. L. (1988). Informed consent and provider–patient relationships in rehabilitation medicine. *Archives of Physical Medicine and Rehabilitation, 69,* 312–317.

Caplan, A. L., Callahan, D., & Haas, J. (1987). Ethical and policy issues in rehabilitation medicine. *Hastings Center Report, 17,* Special Suppl., 1–20.

Childress, J. (1990). The place of autonomy in bioethics. *Hastings Center Report, 17,* 12–17.

Cicerone, K. D. (1989). Psychotherapeutic interventions with traumatically brain-injured patients. *Rehabilitation Psychology, 34,* 105–114.

Davies, J. M. (1996). Dissociation, repression and reality in the countertransference. *Psychoanalytic Dialogues, 6,* 189–218.

Davies, J. M., & Frawley, M. (1994). *Treating adult survivors of childhood sexual abuse.* New York: Basic Books.

Dresser, R., & Whitehouse, P. J. (1994). The incompetent patient on the slippery slope. *Hastings Center Report, 24,* 6–12.

Elliott, C. (1997). Caring about risks: Are severely depressed patients competent to consent to treatment? *Archives of General Psychiatry, 54,* 113–116.

Emanuel, E. J. (1987). A communal vision of care for incompetent patients. *Hastings Center Report, 17,* 15–20.

Felce, D., & Perry, J. (1996). Assessment of quality of life. In R. L. Schalock (Ed.), *Quality of life: Conceptualization and measurement* (Vol. 1; pp. 63–72). Washington, DC: American Association on Mental Retardation.

Fiscalini, J. (1995). The clinical analysis of transference. In M. Lionells, J. Fiscalini, C. H. Mann, & D. B. Stern (Eds.), *The handbook of interpersonal psychoanalysis* (pp. 603–616). Hillsdale, NJ: Analytic Press.

Freedman, M., Stuss, D. T., & Gordon, M. (1991). Assessment of neuropsychological deficits. *Annals of Internal Medicine, 115,* 203–208.

Gabbard, G. O. (1995). Countertransference: The emerging ground. *International Journal of Psycho-Analysis, 76,* 475–485.

Gans, J. S. (1983). Hate in the rehabilitation setting. *Archives of Physical Medicine and Rehabilitation, 64,* 176–179.

Gass, C., & Brown, M. C. (1992). Neuropsychological test feedback to patients with brain dysfunction. *Psychological Assessment, 4,* 272–277.

Gordon, R. M., with Aron, L., Mitchell, S., & Davies, J. M. (1998). Relational psychoanalysis. In R. Langs (Ed.), *Current theories of psychoanalysis* (pp. 31–58). Madison, CT: International Universities Press.

Gunther, M. S. (1987). Catastrophic illness and the caregivers: Real burdens and solutions with respect to the role of the behavioral sciences. In B. Caplan (Ed.), *The rehabilitation desk reference* (pp. 219–243). Rockville, MD: Aspen.

Haas, J. (1987). Ethical considerations of goal setting for patient care in rehabilitation medicine. *American Journal of Physical Medicine and Rehabilitation, 72,* 312–317.

Haffey, W. J. (1989). The assessment of clinical competency to consent to medical rehabilitation interventions. *Journal of Head Trauma Rehabilitation, 4,* 43–56.

Hoffman, I. Z. (1983). The patient as interpreter of the analyst's experience. *Contemporary Psychoanalysis, 19,* 389–422.

Hoffman, I. Z. (1991). Discussion: Toward a social-constructivistic view of the analytic situation. *Psychoanalytic Dialogues, 1,* 74–105.

Hoffman, I. Z. (1992). Some practical implications of a social-constructivistic view of the analytic situation. *Psychoanalytic Dialogues, 2,* 287–304.

Holmes, J. (1996). Values in psychotherapy. *American Journal of Psychotherapy, 50,* 259–273.

Hughes, C., & Hwang, B. (1996). Attempting to conceptualize and measure quality of life. In R. L. Schalock (Ed.), *Quality of life: Conceptualization and measurement* (Vol. 1; pp. 51–62). Washington, DC: American Association on Mental Retardation.

Jennings, B. (1993). Healing the self: The moral meanings of relationships in rehabilitation. *American Journal of Physical Medicine and Rehabilitation, 72,* 401–404.

Kirschner, K. L. (1995). Changing models for the health care provider-patient relationship. *Topics in Stroke Rehabilitation, 2,* 78–79.

Knapp, H. D. (1988). Projective identification: Whose projection—whose identification? *Psychoanalytic Psychology, 6,* 47–58.

Langer, K. G. (1992). Psychotherapy with the neuropsychologically impaired adult. *American Journal of Psychotherapy, 46,* 620–639.

Langer, K. G., & Padrone, F. J. (1992). Psychotherapeutic treatment of awareness in acute rehabilitation of traumatic brain injury. *Neuropsychological Rehabilitation, 2,* 59–70.

Malec, J. F. (1993). Ethics in brain injury rehabilitation: Existential choices among western cultural beliefs. *Brain Injury, 7,* 383–400.

Marson, D. C., Schmitt, F. A., Ingram, K. K., & Harrell, L. E. (1994). Determining the competency of Alzheimer's patients to consent to treatment and research. *Alzheimer's Disease and Associated Disorders, 8,* 5–10.

Mitchell, S. (1993). *Hope and dread in psychoanalysis.* New York: Basic Books.

Mitchell, S. A. (1997). *Influence and autonomy in psychoanalysis.* Hillsdale, NJ: Analytic Press.

Ogden, T. (1979). On projective identification. *International Journal of Psychoanalysis, 60,* 357–373.

Purtillo, R. (1988). Ethical issues in teamwork: The context of rehabilitation. *Archives of Physical Medicine and Rehabilitation, 69,* 318–322.

Reidy, K., Crozier, K. S., Caplan, B., Kutys, M., & Sinnott, M. C. (1992). Treatment refusals during rehabilitation: Ethical concerns of the interdisciplinary team. *Spinal Cord Injury Psychosocial Process, 5,* 44–51.

Romano, M. D. (1989). Ethical issues and families of brain-injured persons. *Journal of Head Trauma Rehabilitation, 4,* 33–41.

Roth, L., Meisel, A., & Lidz, C. (1977). Tests of competency to consent to treatment. *American Journal of Psychiatry, 134,* 279–284.

Siegler, M. (1993). Falling off the pedestal: What is happening to the traditional doctor-patient relationship? *Mayo Clinic Proceedings, 68,* 461–467.

Stern, D. B. (1996). Dissociation and constructivism: Commentary on papers by Davies and Harris. *Psychoanalytic Dialogues, 6,* 252–266.

Stern, D. B. (1997). *Unformulated experience: From dissociation to imagination in psychoanalysis.* Hillsdale, NJ: Analytic Press.

Venesy, B. A. (1994). A clinician's guide to decision making capacity and ethically sound medical decisions. *American Journal of Physical Medicine and Rehabilitation, 73,* 219–226.

Wegener, S. T. (1996). The rehabilitation ethic and ethics. *Rehabilitation Psychology, 41,* 5–17.

PART II

Emotional Factors and Defensive Functioning: Diagnostic and Conceptual Issues in Treatment

4.

Awareness and Denial in Psychotherapy

Karen G. Langer, Ph.D.

The phenomenon of unawareness in brain dysfunction is intriguing at a theoretical level, and challenging at a clinical level. The finding that a patient after brain injury or stroke may actually be, at some level, unaware of some or all of the physical or neuropsychological changes, let alone of their implications, is often startling to the clinician who witnesses this.

Of course, in standard psychiatric and psychotherapy practice, it is not unusual to view the phenomenon of emotional denial among the defense mechanisms, and to attempt to understand its role in shaping personality and in influencing behavior.

Emotional denial may cloud conscious awareness of aspects of reality, certainly at the level of affect, so that the person is not aware of the underlying psychic processes that are operating or guiding his or her activity (including thoughts and feelings). Of course, these processes are inferred or indirectly observed.

In this chapter, we consider the operations of emotional denial along with those of disruptions of brain functioning after brain injury or stroke, in order to understand better the diagnostic and psychotherapeutic challenges of these operations. What is striking about unawareness of disability in brain

injury is the sharp and dramatic contrast of the patient's interpretations (of what is wrong) with the quite visible physical
losses and notable limitations. In extreme form, a patient with
right hemisphere dysfunction on an inpatient unit may actually
"deny" or disavow that the paralyzed left arm is his or hers,
and state that it is someone else's. One of our patients actually
asked her husband to get his hand off her bed, and struggled
with her unimpaired hand to push her own paralyzed arm off
the bed, to her husband's horror. Patients with hemianopsia
may state that they "see just fine" or simply need new glasses.
One patient read a hallway sign advertising a spring raffle, and
asked with puzzlement, "What is a ring affle"; another patient,
equally puzzled, inquired about "feteria" (cafeteria), but without a sense that there was something wrong with his visual
perception. Unawareness of disability in different patient samples with brain impairment including traumatic brain injury
and stroke is amply reviewed (Blonder & Ranseen, 1994; Levine, 1990; McGlynn & Schacter, 1989; Prigatano & Schacter,
1991). This paper focuses on the psychodiagnostic and psychotherapeutic implications of unawareness and denial in patients
with brain injury and stroke.

The question we naturally ask ourselves when witnessing a
graphic display of unawareness, with the patient behaving *as if*
there is no problem, is *how* can the person *not know* about this,
how can she or he not *realize?* And the word *realize* is a key to
beginning the exploration of the nature of unawareness.

Some fundamental questions become apparent to anyone
studying the phenomena of unawareness and denial, with implications for studies of brain function, psychic functioning,
psychopathology, cognitive processing, and consciousness;
these include:

1. What is the **source** or **etiology of unawareness?** This
question is basically diagnostic in nature, and is fundamental
to our scientific method of inquiry and treatment, since there
may be differential treatment efficacy depending on the etiology.

2. What is the **content** of awareness being considered, that
is, awareness of what? This question may often be clouded when
terms such as **awareness of disability,** of **condition** or **illness,** of

prognosis, or of **affect,** among others, are used interchangeably, or without any distinction at all. Patients may often know about the diagnosis of stroke or head injury and even the symptoms, but not of the implications or prognosis. This lack of knowledge may be due to naiveté and/or lack of medical sophistication, or to defensive denial, so the assumption that awareness of prognosis is a natural corollary of the awareness of condition may be inaccurate.

3. **How much** awareness does the patient have: full, partial, or none? Some patients may be fully aware, but others may have only partial or implicit knowledge of deficits so that they may verbally deny the deficit, but their behavior or other communication suggests that they do have *implicit* knowledge (Kihlstrom & Tobias, 1991; Schacter & Prigatano, 1991).

One may also wonder whether awareness after brain dysfunction is any different from denial of disability after other medical illnesses-disabilities, which we know is not uncommon (for discussion, see reviews in Caplan & Schechter, 1987; Langer, 1994; Lewis, 1991). The relationship between depression and awareness or denial is also of interest (Folks, Freeman, Sokol, & Thurstin, 1988; Havik & Maeland, 1986). These issues are also being addressed in clinical studies at the Rusk Institute.

The work of writers including Gazzaniga (Gazzaniga, 1970; Gazzaniga & LeDoux, 1978), Kihlstrom (Kihlstrom & Tobias, 1991), and Hilgard (1977), among others, offer fascinating insights into mechanisms of conscious awareness, for those interested in exploring the subject in greater depth.

DEFENSE MECHANISMS AND AWARENESS IN BRAIN DYSFUNCTION

The need of the psyche to protect itself from threat is the key to the deployment of the defenses. In her influential work on the ego and defense mechanisms, Anna Freud (1936/1966) distinguishes repression as a defense against instinctual drives (i.e., the ego defending against itself) from the defense of denial against an external reality or knowledge. She suggests that without the protection of the defense-in-place, anxiety can overwhelm the ego, and symptoms may overtake adjustment.

This model of defense mechanisms, which helps to explain emotional contributants to unawareness, presupposes that the psyche recognizes at some fundamental level that the information is noxious or threatening to its own integrity. The defense is employed purposefully, then, although the threat itself may be only vaguely perceived, or even unconscious.

Useful conceptualizations of unawareness and denial have focused on the adaptiveness of defense and the degree of distortion of reality. Breznitz (1983) has defined awareness in terms of levels of increasing distortion, including denial of information, threat, personal relevance, urgency, vulnerability, responsibility, affect, and affect relevance. Janis (1983) differentiates adaptive and pathological denial, along with an intermediate "pathogenic denial" that involves minimization of threat, but without a break with reality.

Classic psychologic defense mechanisms may mimic in content the neurologic forms of unawareness or anosagnosia (meaning unawareness of deficit), and vice versa. Each of the statements below could be made in the defense of the ego, by preventing conscious awareness of painful loss or diminishment. Alternatively, they might not have ego-defensive purpose, but reflect a cognitively based inability to understand or appreciate what has happened. For example, the statement, "I have no problem" could be emotional denial; "At my age, we all forget," could be projection (and not just a faulty interpretation); "I am just too tired to read because it is late in the day," could be rationalization; "It's difficulty with vision (visual acuity), not my concentration-memory that's the problem," could be displacement; or "My memory is better now than it was before," could be reaction formation. In other words, the same statement may reflect either faulty interpretation due to cognitive dysfunction (in the case of unawareness), or the actions of the defense mechanisms.

We should remember that denial, when operating as a defense mechanism, is indeed always nonconscious. The purposefulness of the defense is in contradistinction with its nonconscious, nonvolitional operation. People are not conscious of using the defense of denial themselves when they do, but others around them may readily recognize the operation of this defense. Of course, this can be very frustrating for the observer.

With regard to the emotional–defensive source of unawareness, reasons the psyche gives for the existence of the problem are designed to protect the person from threat and anxiety associated with conscious attention to the underlying problem.

On the other hand, in brain dysfunction, neuropsychologic deficits may themselves interfere with a patient's ability to become aware of limitations, disability, loss, or implications. The deficits may also disrupt the self-appraisal and self-monitoring skills needed to be sensitive to the impact on others of speech, behavior, or disability. Neuropsychologic functions that may have significant impact on awareness include: (1) arousal; (2) mental status; (3) thought quality (coherence, logic, concreteness, flexibility-rigidity, conceptual judgment, ability to prioritize and categorize); (4) attention and distractibility; (5) memory (all forms); (6) ability to learn, plan, and anticipate consequences; (7) ability to process emotions (of self and others); and (8) egocentricity and ability to take another's point of view.

Prigatano (1996) has provided one of the most helpful distinctions between the phenomena of unawareness and denial in brain impairment. He explains that denial "represents an attempt to cope; in contrast, impaired self-awareness simply reflects a failure to recognize a need to cope" (p. 200).

MODELS OF UNAWARENESS

Historically, the phenomenon of unawareness of deficit accompanying brain dysfunction has been approached from a number of vantage points. Traditionally, unawareness has been considered a neurologic feature or actual symptom of certain cerebral lesions, particularly of the nondominant hemisphere. *Anosagnosia* was the term first used by the neurologist Babinski in 1914 to describe unawareness of deficit after neurologic insult. Motivational factors and emotional implications were later introduced as explanations of the phenomenon (Weinstein & Kahn, 1955), such that denial of the deficit was considered to be related to premorbid high expectations of the self, which would no longer be viable and would therefore be intolerable. Weinstein has revised the neuropsychiatric approach to denial and unawareness, adding to the motivational and adaptive components the importance of networks involving cortical, limbic, and paralimbic connections and interhemispheric relations (Weinstein, 1991), as well as of personality factors and even cultural influences (citing the work of Gainotti in 1975). Weinstein states that "the existence and form of denial/anosagnosia are determined by the location and rate of development of the brain lesion, the situation in which the denial is elicited, the type of disability, and the way the patient perceives its meaning on the basis of his past experience" (p. 254).

Recent literature describes the development of several sophisticated neurogenic models to explain the phenomenon of unawareness; these point to disrupted neuropsychologic functioning as a cause of unawareness of deficit. Bisiach and colleagues (Bisiach, Valler, Perani, Papagno, & Berti, 1986) propose a modality-specific unawareness, related to particular lesion sites, with each sensory modality (such as hearing, vision, etc.) having its own self-contained, individual awareness. In this model, awareness of one deficit may exist without awareness of the other. In contrast, McGlynn and Schacter (1989) posit that unawareness is independent, and has its own systemic mechanism (the conscious awareness system), which is interconnected to all specific modalities, so that either the system itself or the interconnections may be disrupted. In fact, a book has been devoted entirely to various theoretical and clinical explanations of awareness of deficit after brain injury, with contributions by a number of prominent writers (edited by Prigatano & Schacter, 1991).

Levine (1990) has proposed that unawareness is the immediate fundamental result of sensory deficits at any level, and that there is "no immediate sensory experience that uniquely specifies the deficit . . . sensory loss must be *discovered* by a process of self-observation and inference . . . no information . . .

specifies the absence of a sensory stimulus" (p. 233). He suggests that cognitive impairment is a necessary condition for unawareness, but only for certain easily discovered deficits such as acquired blindness, and not for the harder to discover deficits such as left visual inattention.

Our model at New York University represented an attempt to integrate the psychological and dynamic factors that may play a role in certain patients who display unawareness, with the neuropsychologic or cognitive ingredients of conscious awareness.

The tripartite model, as we call it, has three components, called **information, implication,** and **integration** (Langer & Padrone, 1992). The first source of not knowing, or not being aware, may simply involve not having the information or data. (Levine has discussed the neurologic perspective on discovering information.) The patient may lack the **information,** or lack the technical expertise or medical sophistication to understand the meaning of the information, and/or may have anosagnosia as a neurologic symptom. The second source of not knowing involves **implication,** where someone has the information but may not be able to glean the implications. At the level of unawareness, the patient cannot take "self-as-object" (and may have difficulty with an abstract attitude of self-reflection), or cannot understand the information (whether linguistically or cognitively), or cannot retain or recall the information, or has insufficient arousal for awareness. At the level of minimization, the patient has the information but cannot understand or abstract from the information its consequences and implications (impaired "if/then" processing), so these are minimized. The third source of not knowing involves emotional **integration**. The person has the information and knows the problem, but cannot tolerate the full impact of the information emotionally, so she or he "makes light" of it, at the level of minimization. At the level of denial, the person cannot believe the information because it is too stressful, painful, shocking, or overwhelming; the information is held at bay from conscious experience, or the person's words or actions suggest that she or he does not or cannot believe it and does not integrate it. This denial is typical when the truth is really shocking or when the news is catastrophic.

NEUROGENIC VERSUS EMOTIONAL SOURCES OF UNAWARENESS

In our clinical practice, we are often faced with the question of the complex interplay between contributions of neurogenic causes of unawareness versus those of emotional factors. Careful assessment of the causes of unawareness, or consideration of the possible interaction of causes, is crucial in maximizing the effectiveness of treatment and in enhancing the patient's response. Just as treating a neuropsychological deficit as emotionally based may be destructive to the patient's psyche, aside from being ineffective (Langer, 1992; Lewis & Rosenberg, 1990; Prigatano et al., 1986; Prigatano, 1991), so is the converse, that is, treating denial as a neurologically based unawareness. To make matters more difficult, a patient can be found to "know" about a deficit at one moment, and to seemingly "not know" the next, and we are left to figure out whether this means that the patient had only a transient cognitive appreciation to begin with (Langer & Padrone, 1992), or whether she or he is showing a form of the natural variability in denial (Horowitz, 1983). We realize that our challenge is compounded because we know that sources of not knowing may *coexist,* with both the neuropsychological and the emotional features operating at the same time, so we have recommended the consideration of multiple meanings of not knowing in a given patient, which is similar to the psychoanalytic concept of "multiple determination" (Hartmann, 1939/1958).

Signs and symptoms of emotional denial that will help the clinician to identify it include: the avoidance of associational connections or continuity of meaning; a reduced level of expected emotional responsiveness and emotional numbness or constriction; disavowal of meanings of stimuli; and loss of appropriate reality or fantasies that counteract reality (Horowitz, 1983, p. 134).

But there are also some other clues that may help us to distinguish emotional denial from cognitive unawareness:

1. By definition, denial as a defense serves a need; it protects from psychic threat. Can one detect a need or a threat that would potentially foster the defensive use of denial?
2. What are the cognitive or neuropsychological limitations of the patient? Could these compromise awareness?
3. What happens when the patient is:
   a. Given information?
   b. Confronted about the deficit?
   c. Offered strategies to compensate for the cognitive difficulties that impede awareness?

We would expect that emotional denial, when provided with information, would show no resolution. In fact, cognitive remediation and review of neuropsychological deficits might result in resistance or even, potentially, decompensation. Indeed, if the patient responds best to treating the resistance first, or the threat, it is probably an emotional denial. On the other hand, for a neuropsychologically based deficit, the patient may show response to education and cognitive remediation.

Certain predictions regarding denial and unawareness have been generated from our clinical conceptualizations (Langer & Padrone, 1992). First, the more acute the onset (i.e., recent), the more likely there will be unawareness (due at least in part to the information issue). Second, the worse the cognitive deficit, the more likely that there may be some unawareness (due to a neuropsychological difficulty). Third, the greater the premorbid tendency to use denial or repression as defenses, especially with greater subjective loss, the more likely we would be to predict unawareness, although there may be much interindividual variability. (This may also help explain why some patients deny and others do not.) Fourth, the greater the emotional denial, the less the manifest depression, although this is not absolute (and it is not necessarily true that the less the denial, the greater the depression); there may also be selective denial.

CASE EXAMPLES

With these clues in mind to help us, we present the examples below to illustrate our attempt to distinguish between emotional denial and neuropsychologically based unawareness.

Case 1

The following is a transcript from an initial evaluation of a 74-year-old woman with posterior left hemisphere brain injury after hitting head in a fall on the ice (with surgical evacuation of left temporoparietal subdural hematoma).

In this transcript we will see the minor role of cognitive factors relative to what begins to emerge as the very strong impact of emotional denial on her awareness of disability. There were clear historical roots of the defense of denial that emerged in later psychotherapy.

E: What happened to bring you here?
P: I don't know.
E: So you have no idea why you are here?
P: No, not at all, I don't know why I'm here.
E: Well, tell me what the problem was in the first place.
P: My kids seem to think that when I want to say a word, another word comes out, close to what I mean, I think, in talking.
E: You look sort of sad right now.
P: Because they think I talk wrong.
E: And you don't?
P: I don't.
E: Well, why is it that you are sitting in a wheelchair?
P: I don't know, maybe because they, the nurses, say you have to use it in rehabilitation, and because they said I

once came to class without it and they said I have to use it.

E: Well, are your legs weak at all?

P: No. Maybe they said it because they think I walked to the left, and then another time, to the right.

E: How about your arms, is either arm weak?

P: The left. Because of my surgery on my brain. {Patient has right hemiparesis}.

E: You know, you just said the left.

P: I did? Well, see [what I mean].

E: Yes. So is it the left or the right?

P: I meant the right.

E: You said surgery. Why did you need it?

P: I had bleeding in my head.

E: How did you know you had it?

P: I fell.

E: When was this?

P: November, no, October 1994.

E: How were the symptoms then?

P: Well, first not too much, just a headache; but 2 years, no, 2 weeks later, they did an MRI; then they did see something, and they sent me to a neurosurgeon.

E: Where did he operate?

P: Over here (patient points correctly to the left side of head). That's why I have no hair there. That's it.

E: So why *are* you here now?

P: For occupational therapy, and other, whatever it's called.

E: Well, what's the purpose of being here?

P: To get on my feet more, to start to *not* walk to one side.

E: I'm curious, before you said you had no idea why you were here, and now you give very clear reasons for being here.

P: I look at it as nothing, but it [really] is something.

E: So it sounds like you make light of it?

P: I do [smile].

In this vignette, we observe the patient's tendency to defensively deny, avoid, or minimize her disability. What was compelling in the psychotherapy treatment, and added to the data in favor of the denial hypothesis, were the obvious historical roots of the patient's denial that emerged as a premorbid style of response to stress. The patient noted in therapy, once her tendency to make light of disability was illustrated to her, that this had been a lifelong coping technique, one that she believed she needed to employ to deal with her husband's infidelity for many years. She quite literally drew her attention away from its significance as she stewed in a repressed, quiet rage and hurt.

Our second example illustrates the prominence of unawareness secondary to significant cognitive dysfunction, including short-term memory difficulties and confusion, in a man of superior intellect and achievement.

Case 2

The following is a transcript of an interview with a 77-year-old man with closed head injury due to motor vehicle accident sustained while suffering a heart attack.

E: What happened to bring you here?

P: I'm just here for entertainment; I have no real problem.

E: I'm not sure I know what you mean.

P: I thought all these programs were designed for patients at the hospital so that they could learn something to stimulate their minds; somehow I forgot for the moment that it's a hospital and I considered it like a hotel, like the Concord, like the psychologist has a forum at 2 P.M., and then I remembered that it's a hospital.

E: Well, what was the problem that brought you here first?

P: I had a heart attack a couple of weeks ago, in a car crash.

E: Do you remember it?

P: My wife remembers it better; she's the observer.

E: How is your memory now?

P: I feel like Keats said, {patient quotes accurately from *Ode to a Nightingale*}; we read it repetitively in college, then I got a C.P.A., from there to the army in World War II.

E: I see; tell me, what was your rank?

P: I went from a private to a corporal, to DOD (sic), to the army; I don't know if you understand. After the corporal, my case, in Detroit, it was Louisiana at the beginning, the army . . . the Atomic Bomb, I'll tell you quickly. . . .

E: Let's return to more recent times. Can you tell me what exactly is the purpose of being a patient here now?

P: I said before, I had nothing to do. What time is it?

The patient's confusion and fluctuating attention are glaringly apparent in this case, although certainly emotional factors may also have shaped his interactional style.

Other examples of cognitively based unawareness that have some obvious bases in neuropsychological impairment, with relatively little apparent role of emotional denial, follow.

Case 3

The following is a transcript of an interview with a 60-year-old-man, with a doctorate in biophysics, with stroke due to left frontal hemorrhage.

E: What happened to bring you here?

P: I thought about it. I looked around but it didn't make sense. Something happened between my wife and me; there was some CIA work; I would go into government, but I am too old for starting a new job. My wife suddenly took ill. My science teeters in and out and I have to rely on what other people tell me. I put in an application to the CIA and they asked both of us to come see them. I am not sure if it was that occasion that the vehicle we were driving had an accident with another vehicle, a CIA truck.

E: Why are you in the hospital now?

P: Well, I am in the hospital because my wife in that accident had a severe sprain of the right ankle and hand that worsened and needed a continuous therapy process . . .

E:　And you are here because?

P:　Because the sprain won't heal and the atomic (sic) is very slow in healing.

In the next vignette, a patient with a right hemisphere stroke who was aware of physical but not cognitive limitations, who was disoriented to time, and only grossly oriented to place, tried to make sense out of her disability in the face of some memory loss and confusion. She had a left visual field defect and hemisensory loss in addition to the hemiplegia. (She had been informed that she had sustained a stroke.) There was no denial of affect, as the patient readily discussed her depression and emotional reactions to loss and limitation.

Case 4

The following is a transcript of an interview with a 50-year-old woman with right hemisphere stroke.

E:　What happened to bring you to the hospital?

P:　I broke my arm and leg.

E:　Did someone tell you that?

P:　No, no one told me. I think I remember falling. My husband drove me to the hospital, I think. I really don't remember.

E:　Have you noticed any trouble with your memory lately?

P:　Oh no, clear as a bell as they say.

E:　What have the doctors told you about your arm and leg?

P:　That they are broken and it will take about a year for them to heal; for me a year feels like forever.

E:　That is certainly understandable. It's hard to just wait.

P:　It feels awful for me. My son is a doctor here you know.

E:　What kind of doctor?

P:　I can't really remember. His name is John. I have two other sons; Bill and Tom (sic; there are really four sons). Anyway my son says I will be better soon.

E: So why are you here with us now?
P: I'm here so my bones can heal. I broke my foot once before, or was it my arm? Well, I broke something once before and couldn't use it for a while. It's just so frustrating. I also hate being so dependent. Do you see that piece of trash on the floor? Normally I would just pick it up myself. I hate being so dependent. . . . And to boot they are having me see a psychologist this morning.
E: That's me.
P: Oh, well you're very nice, so that's O.K. (She laughed).

Our next vignette illustrates the dual and simultaneous contributions of unawareness (due to informational and cognitive factors) with a defensive style that fostered denial.

Case 5

The following is a transcript of a psychotherapy session with a 48-year-old woman with stroke due to a right frontal subarachnoid hemorrhage and clipping of anterior communicating artery aneurysm.

P: You know, I slept at home last night in my own bed (Note: this is inaccurate; patient was a hospital inpatient).
E: Tell me what you need to gain from being back here in the rehabilitation center then today.
P: Nothing. I always use a shopping cart, and I only cook for one so I have no heavy oven trays to carry. So what do I need? A cleaning girl (smiles).
E: Well, do you have any goals in being here?
P: To find a husband (smiling). I don't know. I'm here to get better. I want to walk, to get better, and to lead a normal life.
E: What exactly is disrupted at this time?
P: The hospital controls the situation; I'm don't act on my own.

E: If you left today, is there anything that would be hard
       for you to do?

P: To find a salad for dinner (smiling). Really, the ordinary
       routines of life, it's all done for you, they wash and
       dress you.

E: Is there anything difficult since the aneurysm for which
       you need help?

P: No.

E: Are there any physical changes now?

P: Yes, I have to get the sphincter muscle in order; I get
       wet.

E: Oh, that can be difficult and pretty embarrassing. Well,
       it seems that there is a goal that you can work on improv-
       ing while you are here. I notice that you sit in a wheel-
       chair. Why is that?

P: They [the nurses] put you there.

E: Why is that?

P: They don't want you to move about; they're worried
       that you might fall and break your back and sue.

E: Why would they be more worried about that now?

P: You don't have the balance.

E: So you're aware of the balance.

P: I guess so. It's a genuine fear. Do you sway and act
       drunk and waver when you walk?

E: Well, was that ever a problem before the aneurysm?

P: It may have been. I have a short memory; that's a lit-
       tle problem.

E: Isn't that something you would like then to work on im-
       proving?

P: It's a goal; so you've given me a goal (smiling).

E: How is the strength in your legs; any weaker recently?

P: No, it was all prior, from arthritis.

E: How about concentration and memory; are they
       harder?

P: No, nothing since the aneurysm has changed, I had
       ADD—you know, attention deficit disorder; I always had
       trouble concentrating.

E: But the balance?

P: I never really had balance.

E: You're saying there are no changes since the aneurysm?
P: Well, there are some changes that I have to work on.
E: What are they?
P: Balance, concentration.
E: So you feel that you should be here?
P: Absolutely. I need therapy for walking; there are no side effects of the stroke, but I guess I forget this and that.
E: So your goals are walking, balance, concentration, and memory. How come, though, at the beginning you didn't mention these?
P: Maybe I'm more resilient now, or more trusting of you. Maybe I was protecting myself.

The interaction of emotional denial and cognitively based unawareness are readily apparent here.

ASSESSMENT ISSUES

In order to treat a patient most effectively, we need to accurately assess a broad range of aspects of life-functioning and psychologic adaptation.

There are formal questionnaires that can be used to assess awareness of disability after brain dysfunction (Prigatano et al., 1986; Simon, Riley, Egelko, Kaplan, Newman, & Diller, 1991). For the patient with questionable awareness, one may inquire, with increasing structure and specificity, about circumstances of onset, name, and nature of the condition, other health problems, the nature of the disability (both physical and cognitive), the degree of dependence and assistance needed, expectations of self and others, and goals for treatment, with examples of queries contained in the vignettes presented above.

TREATMENT IMPLICATIONS

There are some treatment implications that emerge. If a neuropsychological (implication) difficulty is what obscures knowledge and awareness, the clinician should work on building *cognitive structures* that would support the knowledge. If, on the other hand, emotional denial predominates, then the therapeutic effort would instead best focus on strengthening the *ego functions* that could support the knowledge. (The two possibilities are of course not mutually exclusive, and if the stress produces regression in ego functioning, structure, support, and reeducation may be needed until psychic equilibrium is restored.)

There are some other therapeutic considerations in treating either unawareness or denial. We need to balance the risk of despair, versus the need to maintain hope; the risk of shame, versus the need to maintain self-esteem and self-respect; the risk of psychic decompensation were the denial to be punctured; and the nature and level of distress and the patient's ability to tolerate it. The risks involved in maintaining denial or unawareness, though, may include real physical danger to self or others if the patient ignores the physical reality (and tries to climb out of bed or drive a car, for example), or may be emotional if the patient risks failure and humiliation that could have been otherwise averted. Of course, the positive side to denial is that, certainly in the acute phases, it may permit adaptive coping with catastrophic loss. It may also fuel creative endeavor that would be impossible if the patient became fully resigned to a sense of limitation as opposed to one of challenge.

In psychotherapeutic treatment of awareness (whether cognitively based or emotionally driven), the *therapeutic alliance* is paramount for the patient to feel secure and trusting. There may be a tendency to get to the point quickly and uncover all the difficulties, but *prioritization* and *hierarchy* must take precedence if the patient is to feel a sense that she or he can tackle the problem. Lewis (1991) cautions wisely that denial "is not an obstacle to treatment to be overcome as quickly as possible but rather, as a motivated process that has adaptive value and meaning" (p. 235), and although adaptive, it is not maintained without a price.

Clinical strategies with which we are all familiar include *dosing or titration* of the painful information at a pace that can be tolerated, effectiveness and *sensitivity of timing,* and *empathic tone* and wording. The use of *humor* can make a real difference in lightening the tone of difficult topics, and can help the patient consolidate the new awareness with an emotional frame, one that decreases the dread of isolation and shares what is fundamentally human in the therapist as well. Another key factor in addressing awareness is the patient's perception of the direct *relevance* to him or her, as well as the *premorbid context and meaning* of the loss. This involves considerations of the normal narcissistic aspects of the patient's self-image. Cicerone (1998) sensitively discusses the importance of consideration of the patient's assumptions and beliefs about his or her own world, calling for real therapeutic neutrality and a nonjudgmental stance. The therapist needs to continuously monitor current and potential sources of distress to titrate these, and to provide support for the shame, hurt, and pain.

To summarize, the psychotherapeutic challenge involves monitoring the dynamic fluctuations in a patient's readiness to become aware of losses, considering the interaction of neurogenic and emotional factors, and sensitivity to and therapeutic treatment of the emotional reactions, such as shame, depression, anger, and/or despair, that may accompany growing awareness of loss. We as therapists ought also to consider the importance of maintaining (realistic) optimism and hope (Janis & Mann, 1977) that change is possible and that patients can find ways to live with loss and to overcome certain obstacles. This determination is not akin to denial, for in it the person recognizes the limitation, but is motivated to find ways to adapt and live with it. Lastly, we remind ourselves of our own humanity, particularly when dealing with patients with brain dysfunction when we work on awareness, since we realize that many of us have pockets of diminished awareness of our being, or of our own strengths and weaknesses, undesirable in certain instances but adaptive in others. But building conscious awareness is after all a hallmark of the challenge that we all face as individuals in our own continued development.

REFERENCES

Babinski, J. (1914). Contribution a l'etude des troubles mentaux dans l'hemiplegie organique cerebrale (anosagnosie). (Contribution to the study of mental troubles in organic cerebral hemiplegia [anosagnosia]). *Revue Neurologique (Paris), 22,* 845–848.

Bisiach, E., Valler, G., Perani, D., Papagno, C., & Berti, A. (1986). Unawareness of disease following lesions of the right hemisphere: Anosagnosia for hemiplegia and anosagnosia for hemianopia. *Neuropsychologia, 24,* 471–482.

Blonder, L. X., & Ranseen, J. D. (1994). Awareness of deficit following right hemisphere stroke. *Neuropsychiatry, Neuropsychology, and Behavioral Neurology, 7,* 260–266.

Breznitz, S. (1983). The seven kinds of denial. In S. Breznitz (Ed.), *The denial of stress* (pp. 257–280). New York: International Universities Press.

Caplan, B., & Schechter, J. (1987). Depression and denial in disabling illness. In B. Caplan (Ed.), *Rehabilitation psychology desk reference* (pp. 133–170). Rockville, MD: Aspen.

Cicerone, K. (1998). Psychotherapy throughout the course of recovery from traumatic brain injury. *Brain Injury Source, 1,* 51–53.

Folks, D. G., Freeman, A. M. III, Sokol, R. S., & Thurstin, A. H. (1988). Denial: Predictor of outcome following coronary bypass surgery. *International Journal of Psychiatry in Medicine, 18,* 57–66.

Freud, A. (1966). The ego and the mechanisms of defense. (Rev. ed.). In *The writings of Anna Freud* (Vol. 2). New York: International Universities Press. (Original work published 1936).

Gainotti, G. (1975). Confabulation of denial in senile dementia. *Psychiatria Clinica, 8,* 99–108.

Gazzaniga, M. S. (1970). *The bisected brain.* New York: Appleton-Century-Crofts.

Gazzaniga, M. S., & LeDoux, J. F. (1978). *The integrated mind.* New York: Plenum.

Hartmann, H. (1958). *Ego psychology and the problem of adaptation.* New York: International Universities Press. (Original work published 1939).

Havik, O. E., & Maeland, J. G. (1986). Dimensions of verbal denial in myocardial infarction. *Scandinavian Journal of Psychology, 27,* 326–339.

Hilgard, E. R. (1977). *Divided consciousness: Multiple controls in human thought and action.* New York: Wiley.

Horowitz, M. J. (1983). Psychological response to serious life events. In S. Breznitz (Ed.), *The denial of stress* (pp. 129–159). New York: International Universities Press.

Janis, I. L. (1983). Preventing pathogenic denial by means of stress inoculation. In S. Breznitz (Ed.), *The denial of stress* (pp. 129–159). New York: International Universities Press.

Janis, I. L., & Mann, L. (1977). *Decision making: A psychological analysis of conflict, choice and commitment.* New York: Free Press.

Kihlstrom, J. F., & Tobias, B. A. (1991). Anosagnosia, consciousness, and the self. In G. P. Prigatano & D. L. Schacter (Eds.), *Awareness of deficit after brain injury* (pp. 198–222). New York: Oxford University Press.

Langer, K. G. (1992). Psychotherapy with the neuropsychologically impaired adult. *American Journal of Psychotherapy, 46,* 620–639.

Langer, K. G. (1994). Depression and denial in psychotherapy of persons with disabilities. *American Journal of Psychotherapy, 48,* 181–194.

Langer, K. G., & Padrone, F. J. (1992). Psychotherapeutic treatment of awareness in acute rehabilitation of traumatic brain injury. *Neuropsychological Rehabilitation, 2,* 59–70.

Levine, D. N. (1990). Unawareness of visual and sensorimotor defects: A hypothesis. *Brain and Cognition, 13,* 233–281.

Lewis, L. (1991). Role of psychological factors in disordered awareness. In G. P. Prigatano & D. L. Schacter (Eds.), *Awareness of deficit after brain injury: clinical and theoretical issues* (pp. 223–239). New York: Oxford University Press.

Lewis, L., & Rosenberg, S. J. (1990). Psychoanalytic psychotherapy with brain-injured adult psychiatric patients. *Journal of Nervous and Mental Disease, 178,* 69–77.

McGlynn, S. M., & Schacter, D. L. (1989). Unawareness of deficits in neuropsychological syndromes. *Journal of Clinical and Experimental Neuropsychology, 11,* 143–205.

Prigatano, G. P. (1991). Disordered mind, wounded soul: The emerging role of psychotherapy in rehabilitation after brain injury. *Journal of Head Trauma Rehabilitation, 6,* 1–10.

Prigatano, G. P. (1996). Behavioral limitations TBI patients tend to underestimate: a replication and extension to patients with lateralized cerebral dysfunction. *The Clinical Neuropsychologist, 10,* 191–201.

Prigatano, G., Fordyce, D., Zeiner, H., Roueche, J., Pepping, M., & Wood, B. (1986). *Neuropsychological rehabilitation after brain injury.* Baltimore, MD: Johns Hopkins University Press.

Prigatano, G. P., & Schacter, D. L. (Eds.). (1991). *Awareness of deficit after brain injury.* New York: Oxford University Press.

Schacter, D. L., & Prigatano, G. P. (1991). Forms of unawareness. In G. P. Prigatano & D. L. Schacter (Eds.)., *Awareness of deficit after brain injury* (pp. 258–262). New York: Oxford University Press.

Simon, D., Riley, E., Egelko, S., Kaplan, E., Newman, B., & Diller, L. (1991). *A new instrument for assessing awareness of deficits in stroke.*

Poster presented at the 99th annual convention of the American Psychological Association, San Francisco, CA.

Weinstein, E. A. (1991). Anosagnosia and denial of illness. In G. P. Prigatano & D. L. Schacter (Eds.), *Awareness of deficit after brain injury* (pp. 240–257). New York: Oxford University Press.

Weinstein, E. A., & Kahn, R. L. (1955). *Denial of illness.* Springfield, IL: Charles C Thomas.

5.

Depression and Its Diagnosis and Treatment

Robert W. Butler, Ph.D. and
Paul Satz, Ph.D.

The occurrence of a mood and affective disorder following an injury to the brain is extremely common. The incidence of major depressive disorder following traumatic brain injury (TBI) has been reported to be in the range of 25 to 50% of all patients (Gualtieri & Cox, 1991; Kinsella, Moran, Ford, & Ponsella, 1988; McKinlay, Brooks, Bond, Martinage, & Marshall, 1981). It has also been reported that the severity of the trauma is positively correlated with increased depressed mood following TBI (Satz et al., in press). Similar estimates of frequency have been reported in the stroke population (Robinson & Price, 1982).

Neuropsychologically, the comorbidity of brain impairment and depression can create diagnostic confusion, and make psychological treatment extremely complex. The reasons for this are that many types of brain dysfunction can cause depression symptoms which may exist in the absence of depressed mood. For example, Blumer and Benson (1975) described a syndrome of "pseudodepression" in patients who had suffered damage to the medial and orbital frontal lobes. This syndrome is characterized by apathy, unconcern, a lack of drive, decreased emotionality, and difficulties in the initiation of behaviors. Thus, the patient may present with many of the symptoms of major depressive disorder but not actually manifest the underlying psychiatric disorder. Conversely, major depressive disorder can be characterized by neuropsychological impairment. Patients with major depressive disorder but no discernable central nervous system (CNS) damage have been reported to manifest impairment in attention-concentration, memory (retrieval in particular), and on cognitive tests that require effort (Caine, 1986). *Pseudodementia,* a descriptive term for the presentation of depression with associated cognitive impairment in the elderly, is recognized as a common form of treatable "dementia" (Benson, 1982). Finally, a recent study has suggested the possibility of an interactive relationship between CNS status and the emergence of major depressive disorder. It has been reported that while depression episodes can be characterized by nonverbal intelligence deficits, the pattern of reduced performance IQ, when compared to verbal IQ and with accounting for the timed nature of nonverbal tests, was present in these patients even after the affective disorder remitted (Sackeim et al., 1992).

It is our position that the assessment and treatment of depression in the neurologically impaired patient is not a simple technical process. There is considerable overlap between the symptoms of major depressive disorder without accompanying CNS impairment and the neuropsychological sequelae of a brain injury. Further, depression can be a natural psychological reaction to a neurological disease. Treatment approaches to depression with a neuropsychologically impaired patient will have to take into account additional variables, issues, and factors. In this chapter we will: (1) describe those aspects of depression that are commonly apparent in patients with a primary CNS disorder; (2) offer specific approaches designed to effectively formulate a diagnostic schema for depression in this population; and (3) address important psychotherapeutic issues in the treatment of brain-impaired patients who have a diagnosis of affective disorder.

SYMPTOMS OF DEPRESSION ASSOCIATED WITH NEUROPSYCHOLOGICAL IMPAIRMENT

One of the most common referrals to the clinical neuropsychologist in an adult practice involves a diagnostic question regarding the presence of "pseudodementia." Specifically, the neuropsychologist is asked, "Does this patient suffer from depression, or is a dementing process present?" We believe that this is a specious question, not only in the aged population but also in all differential brain injury/depression diagnostic dilemmas. Rather than asking, "Is the patient depressed or does the individual have a neurological disorder?" one needs to consider, "Is there evidence of depression *and* has the patient suffered a neuropsychological impairment?" The two probabilities are not mutually exclusive. One can be demented and depressed, depressed and not demented, or demented and not depressed. Thus, the diagnostic query is not simple and needs to be multifactorial in nature. In an assessment of depression in the CNS-impaired population the following factors should be entertained.

Mood-Affect

Internal perceptions of emotion can be altered following a brain injury, particularly if the nondominant hemisphere is involved. The ability to perceive emotion in others is associated with posterior nondominant cortical functioning, while the expression of emotionality is more anteriorly located in the nondominant hemisphere (Bryden & Ley, 1983; Heilman, Watson, & Bowers, 1983; Ross, 1981). Behaviorally, the patient with a brain injury can present with incongruent mood and affect due to a defect in the ability to perceive and/or express emotionality. Thus, decreased prosody, absence of gesturing, and a lack of appropriate facial expression secondary to right-sided brain impairment may give the illusion of depression in a patient whose subjective mood is euthymic. The integrity of these and other nondominant hemispheric functions should be directly assessed in a brain-impaired patient who is suspected of having major depressive disorder.

One should also be aware of research evidence which indicates that the presence of depression in a patient with brain impairment can be associated with increased severity of neuropsychological deficits, particularly those of a nondominant nature (Fogel & Sparadeo, 1985). Thus, it is critical that an accurate diagnosis of depression is made and confirmed in a timely manner. Treatment should be instituted rapidly, and neuropsychological functions need to be reevaluated after successful resolution of the affective illness. The neuropsychological evaluation can be an invaluable blueprint for planning rehabilitation efforts, vocational screening, social–marital adjustment counseling, and helping the patient, in general, maximize his or her resources following CNS illness or injury. Misleading neuropsychological results may be present in the patient who is also suffering from a major depressive disorder.

Damage to the frontal lobes and the limbic system can alter emotionality and the expression of affect. This area of the brain is especially prone to contusions following closed head injuries (Gurdjian & Gurdjian, 1976). Thus, a detailed history of past head injuries needs to be obtained on all patients. Frontal damage following a head injury can result in difficulties with initiating behavior, flat affect, impairment in modulating emotion, and excessive lability (Levin, Benton, & Grossman, 1982). These behavioral symptoms can also be expressed by the patient with depression, and it is necessary to identify the underlying causality in order to develop an effective treatment plan.

Neurovegetative Signs

While all of the symptoms of major depressive disorder identified in the *Diagnostic and Statistical Manual* (DSM-IV; APA, 1994) are relevant for a diagnosis, some have decreased sensitivity and specificity in the brain-impaired population. Neurovegetative symptoms, in particular, are less useful for a diagnosis of depression because brain dysfunction can cause alterations in these areas independent of depressed mood. For example, changes in sleep patterns, appetite, energy, memory, arousal, and sex drive can be due to diencephalic and limbic damage secondary to a CNS insult and have reduced diagnostic efficacy (Butler & Satz, 1988; Jorge, Robinson, & Arndt, 1993). A careful review of the time course of symptom emergence will assist the clinician in making a judgment in this area. Neurovegetative symptoms which emerge relatively soon after the brain injury or damage are likely to be less reflective of major depression, particularly if they are not associated with a significant change in mood.

Social/Occupational Functioning

A necessary criterion for the diagnosis of major depressive disorder or another mood disorder is that a significant impairment in social and/or occupational functioning has occurred (APA, 1994). Deficient functioning in these areas is assumed to be secondary to symptoms of depression. Within the brain-impaired population, however, alterations in social and occupational adjustment are very common, even following very subtle cognitive impairment. Denial of illness when combined with neuropsychological impairment can result in decreased vocational performance. Familial and marital relationships often-times undergo stressful upheaval, and the patient may suffer from disabling initiation deficits resulting in social isolation (Butler & Satz, 1988; Lezak, 1978; Prigatano, 1987). Thus, the diagnostic discrimination of these criteria in major depressive disorder with a neuropsychologically dysfunctional patient is reduced.

ASSESSING DEPRESSION IN PATIENTS WITH NEUROPSYCHOLOGICAL IMPAIRMENT

Prior to a clinical assessment for depression with the brain-impaired patient, one will first want to have a detailed history of the neurological insult, review pertinent neurological and neurodiagnostic reports, and obtain a neuropsychological evaluation. This information will provide the clinician with the necessary information required to make an effective diagnosis of mood alterations independent of or associated with CNS impairment. Neurological and neurodiagnostic evaluations will provide evidence of the location, nature, and extent of structural and functional brain damage. A history will allow the clinician to make judgments regarding possible causative relationships between mood, brain dysfunction, and the psychological reaction to CNS illness. The neuropsychological evaluation is an invaluable tool for determining the extent to which occupational and/or social dysfunction is associated with brain impairment, depression, or a combination of both. The importance of this evaluation cannot be overemphasized. A comprehensive neuropsychological evaluation is the only neurodiagnostic procedure that quantifies the end product of brain function: thought and behavior. Quite simply, it is the brain's responsibility to provide the substrate for one's effective and successful adaptation to a complex and demanding world. The neuropsychological evaluation is designed to measure the degree of this role efficacy, which the brain mediates under our conscious activation.

After the neurodiagnostic evaluations have been reviewed and incorporated, the clinician should then determine if a major depressive disorder or dysthymia is present. As noted above, the differential diagnosis of brain impairment versus depression or a "pseudodementia" is somewhat specious. A more clinically relevant and, in our minds, practical approach is to ask first: (1) whether there is evidence of brain dysfunction and (2) whether there is depression present. The assessment of subjective mood is especially critical for a diagnosis of depression in the brain-impaired population. This is because, as identified earlier, the behavioral, affective, and neurocognitive symptoms of depression overlap with many neurobehavioral consequences of brain insults. We strongly recommend using the Beck Scales for Depression as an aide in quantifying mood. The Beck Depression Inventory has been revised (BDI-II: Beck,

Steer, & Brown, 1996) and remains a brief but excellent quanti-fication of depressive mood and ideation. The clinician is also encouraged to supplement the BDI-II with Beck's hopelessness, anxiety, and suicidal ideation scales. These are all very well constructed psychometric measures that provide excellent in-formation on the patient's internal, subjective psychological state. An excellent illustrative example of how these scales can be used clinically with brain-impaired individuals is presented by Hibbard and coworkers (Hibbard, Gordon, Egelko, & Langer, 1987).

While self-report measures of mood are invaluable for identifying dysphoria, they can provide misleading results and should be used with appropriate caution. Most depression in-ventories have been developed using non-brain-impaired pa-tients, and there may be unknown normative discrepancies for this reason. Different rating scales for depression have been demonstrated to have poor concordance for classifying individ-ual "cases" of depression, even though the scales may have very high correlation coefficients with each other (Harker, Satz, D'Elia, Miller, & Jin, 1997). One possible explanation for this discrepancy is that while all self-report measures may be validly assessing depression, some may be more heavily weighted toward the cognitive and neurovegetative aspects of mood disorders (e.g., concentration, memory, fatigue). As noted earlier, these scales can result in increased false positives with neuropsychologically impaired patients. Impaired patients may also have significant perceptual and attentional cognitive deficits that can increase the likelihood of reading errors. Le-sions to the parietal–occipital cortex, and to a lesser extent the temporal lobe, can cause acquired dyslexia (Luria, 1980) which can also reduce the validity of self-report measures with brain-impaired adults and children. Given these caveats, what is needed is a good, thorough clinical assessment using a scien-tific, hypothesis testing approach. The self-report inventory should be closely inspected for each individual item response, in addition to using the summated score for classification. Item responses should be evaluated in light of the clinical interview and verified with the patient if necessary. Any discrepancies between self and family member reporting should also be closely investigated. It is the clinician's responsibility to follow all these steps in order to make an accurate diagnosis.

While the primary focus of this chapter is directed toward the clinician who is treating adults, there are some very important issues specific to the pediatric and adolescent brain-impaired population that should be briefly discussed. The diagnostic criteria for depression in children and adolescents are identical to adults. This should not fool the clinician into thinking that the diagnostic considerations are entirely the same for these two populations. The importance of a comprehensive neuropsychological evaluation, history, and other neurodiagnostic assessments is equally pertinent to the diagnosis of possible depression in brain-impaired children. There are, however, some very critical caveats to differentiating neuropsychological impairment from depressive symptoms in children versus adults. The clinician needs to take into account the status of the child in terms of brain and behavior development. For example, the frontal lobes do not complete myelination and maturation until the second decade of life (Passler, Isaac, & Hynd, 1985). Thus, initiation and self-control difficulties are relatively common in normal children and not necessarily reflective of an actual insult to the frontal brain structures. Further, the status of the child's language development is often a critical factor in assessing mood and in mediating self-control. The child may be unable to accurately label a mood state, or to use internal dialogue in an effective manner.

Child neuropsychology has been emerging as a subdiscipline with its own advanced training requirements. In the case of a brain-impaired child who is suspected of having a mood disorder, the clinician should seek consultation from a professional specifically trained in pediatric neuropsychology. There is a child's version of a self-report depression inventory, The Child Depression Inventory (CDI: Kovacs, 1992). This is a useful measure and should be administered to the patient. While we do not have data to support this impression, in our clinical experience mild elevations on the CDI (T score between 60 or 70) can be suggestive of significant dysphoric mood, especially in a child who is not verbal facile, or who is somewhat delayed or compromised in communication skills. Information on the child's psychological status will also need to be obtained from the caregivers. They can provide critical information on the child's mood and affect, particularly with a patient who is cognitively impaired as well. A clinical interview with the child's caregivers will be illuminating, but this should be supplemented with an other-report psychometric inventory specifically designed to evaluate the presence and severity of a mood disturbance. The two most widely used questionnaires for children and adolescents are the Child Behavior Checklist (CBC: Achenbach, 1991) and the Personality Inventory for Children-Revised (PIC-R: Lachar, 1984). There are advantages to each measure. The CBC is relatively brief but may be somewhat insensitive to mild or moderate dysphoria. This is due, in part, to its brevity, but also because it was constructed to identify clinically significant depression rather than more mild mood dysphorias, such as what would be characteristic of an adjustment disorder. We prefer the PIC-R because of its greater sensitivity and use of validity scales (Butler, Rizzi, & Bandilla, in press). Completing the PIC-R, however, is much more time consuming and requires a cooperative caregiver.

It is very important to note that children, because of brain and language development, often lack the abilities for self-reflection and/or verbal expression of mood alterations. When queried they may fail to endorse corresponding symptoms of depression. Thus, inconsistencies between self-report mood, affect, and behavior are likely to be more prominent in childhood depression. Our clinical experience supports this likelihood, and we believe there are even greater diagnostic problems with neuropsychologically impaired children because language can suffer considerable disruption following a pediatric brain insult. As was noted above, the diagnosis of depression in the neuropsychologically impaired patient necessitates the consideration of additional nuances that will effect the validity and reliability of clinical diagnostic tools. When the patient is a child, even more additional factors must be weighed and analyzed.

PSYCHOTHERAPY OF DEPRESSION WITH
NEUROPSYCHOLOGICALLY IMPAIRED PATIENTS

Over 10 years ago we stated that psychotherapy is just as important of a consideration with the brain-impaired population as it is with cognitively intact individuals (Butler & Satz, 1988). We continue to believe that this is true, and the emergence of this text is a strong indication that others also value the importance of psychotherapy with the patient who has suffered neurological impairment. The traditional belief that these patients could not benefit from insight-oriented, self-exploratory, and/ or cognitively based treatments has not held up over time. Brain-impaired individuals can clearly benefit from these approaches. Psychotherapy with a neuropsychologically impaired person, however, does require special considerations. We will address what we believe to be the most important characteristics of the psychotherapy of depression in brain-impaired patients.

Our primary approach to therapy with both adults and children is cognitive-behavioral. In using this therapeutic approach for depression, the clinician is typically working in two major areas. First, the patient's own self-statements and style of thinking about events in their life, or schemata, are examined. The theoretical assumption is that depressive mood is associated with underlying errors in judgment, and inaccurate or ineffective thought patterns. While the complexity of the internal dialogue will increase with adults as opposed to children, the errors in thinking can be quite similar. Second, the patient's specific behaviors are examined in order to ensure that there is an adequate supply of reinforcers in his or her environment, and that the individual is successfully obtaining rewards in life. Typically, the depressed individual withdraws socially, reduces their access to secondary reinforcers, and will even decrease use of primary reinforcers such as food, and with adults, sexual activity. The patient is given specific homework assignments which are expected to be completed in between psychotherapy sessions. Additionally, the patient is typically required to keep a diary or record of both internal thoughts and behavioral events. The above approaches can be supplemented with direct instruction in coping strategies that are designed to control depressive symptoms, and also social skills training to increase life-style reinforcers, particularly with children and adolescents (Stark, Rouse, & Livingston, 1991).

The reader has probably already identified the neurocognitive deficits that would directly impact on this type of psychotherapy. Cognitive–behavioral therapy for depression requires some degree of initiation, the ability to learn new verbal material, language comprehension and expression skills, memory and attention-concentration. While these neuropsychological functions can suffer some degree of impairment following a brain injury, rarely do they all become profoundly impaired. Even children with severe neuropsychological involvement typically have rudimentary language systems and basic learning abilities. Thus, it is the rare patient who has undergone a serious global or specific neuropsychological deterioration to the degree that they are inappropriate candidates for cognitive–behavioral therapy for depression. To the extent that some degree of impairment is present, however, the clinician will have to make some allowances and treatment adjustments in order to maximize the potential effectiveness of psychotherapy.

If memory is defective, the patient should be instructed in the use of compensatory devices. Treatment sessions should be tape recorded, and the patient should be taught how to use an organizing system, electronic or script-based. The organizing system is recommended because it can serve as both an appointment schedule and a record-keeping diary for the psychotherapy assignments. If memory is severely impaired, the therapist may want to have an assistant provide periodic reminders to the patient about completing homework assignments. If the patient has a friend, partner, or available family member willing to provide memory reminders this can also be instituted. This "personal assistance" is also necessary for patients who have significant initiation difficulties following a frontal brain injury. In addition to compensatory devices, the patient can be taught mnemonic strategies designed to improve memory functioning. For higher functioning individuals, this can be done in the form of bibliotherapy. There are numerous memory improvement books readily available in all large book-stores. With more impaired patients, consultation with a thera-pist skilled in cognitive remediation and rehabilitation will be helpful.

All neuropsychologically impaired patients who begin psy-chotherapy for depression should be evaluated by a psychiatrist for possible medication treatment. In addition to consideration for antidepressant therapy, the physician should weigh the po-tential benefits of stimulants such as Ritalin, Dexedrine, and Cylert. These approaches can be beneficial with brain-impaired patients in two ways. First, they can be useful in improving attentional deficits associated with CNS dysfunction. Second, stimulants may help counter initiation difficulties that the pa-tient may be suffering (Kraus, 1995).

If the patient has not fully adjusted to the life changes associated with the brain impairment, then this should become a treatment goal, in addition to the more traditional cogni-tive–behavioral procedures. As we have written before (But-ler & Satz, 1988), brain injuries can result in a very unique sense of loss. Specifically, the patient is forced to cope with a loss of the psychological self. If one loses sight or an arm or leg, this is a traumatic event that can lead to depression, but the person still possesses their cognitive abilities and basic per-sonality structure. Social, family, and marital relationships may show some initial strain, but generally remain intact. In our experience, the loss of self that can result from neuropsycholog-ical impairment is a much more devastating event, and can be extremely destructive to social and familial support systems. Others have also made these observations (Lewis, Athey, Ey-man, & Saeks, 1992; Lezak, 1978). A willingness to briefly de-tour, at times, from the goals of therapy for symptoms of major depression is essential. The patient may be in need of empathy, understanding, and support for issues more reactive to the brain impairment and his or her losses. If the patient is suffer-ing from highly significant complications in this area, a referral is necessary. The referral network for the clinician treating a brain-impaired patient for depression needs to include a neu-rologist, neuropsychologist (preferably one skilled in psycho-therapy and cognitive remediation with brain-impaired patients), family therapist, psychiatrist, marital therapist, speech pathologist, occupational therapist, and vocational specialist.

The neuropsychological evaluation will provide important data on the manner in which psychotherapy should proceed. If the patient has a decelerated learning curve and/or reduced information processing efficacy, then the therapeutic process will require greater time. The amount of information imparted in any single treatment session will need to be reduced and tailored to the patient's learning ability. If the patient has an aphasia, a speech pathologist needs to be consulted and therapy altered as appropriate. The degree of neuropsychological impairment will give the clinician a good basis for the initial formulation of appropriate treatment goals.

Denial of symptoms, or anosognosia, is very common following a brain injury (Benson, 1994; Prigatano & Schacter, 1991), and presents an obvious set of hurdles for the psychotherapist. The patient, most often an adult, may deny even the most profound cognitive impairment, including deficits in memory, speech, planning, judgment, and attention-concentration. Personality and mood changes may also be steadfastly ignored and disclaimed. Our experience suggests that direct confrontation for anosognosia is rarely helpful and can be damaging to the therapeutic alliance. We prefer to expose the patient to situations which will force him or her to undergo a self-confrontation process. It is the therapist's role to provide a supportive, but insightful environment so that the patient learns from and accepts the self-confrontation. Related to the issue of symptom denial, the therapist will need to carefully weigh psychodynamic interpretations of resistance with patients who have suffered brain impairment. As described previously, a patient may fail to complete homework repeatedly because they have impaired memory. Similarly, an anosognosia neglect syndrome associated with right hemispheric damage may be present, and the patient may deny and refuse to acknowledge cognitive or mood impairment because of the brain injury not because of "unconscious" psychological processes.

Finally, specific attention will likely have to be directed at familial relationships. For the adult this may involve the marital or other partner, and with children the parents will be involved. Family members may react to the patient with feelings of frustration, guilt, depression, resentment, and/or anger (Cooper, 1976; Lezak, 1978). Overinvolvement and intrusive caretaking may begin to occur, or conversely, partners or caretakers may deny the patient's illness and attempt to continue their relationship as if nothing has changed. Delicate role balances in the family relationships that have been established can become extremely disrupted. While the therapist may have recommended, and begun treating the neuropsychologically impaired patient for individual psychotherapy of depression, it is quite probable that family therapy issues will become prominent, especially if a family member has been enlisted as a therapeutic assistant. Referral and treatment by a competent family and/or marital therapist is necessary should these issues arise.

REFERENCES

Achenbach, T. M. (1991). *Manual for the child behavior checklist/4-18 and 1991 profile.* Burlington, VT: University of Vermont Department of Psychiatry.

American Psychiatric Association (1994). *Diagnostic and statistical manual of mental disorders* (4th ed.). Washington, DC: Author.

Beck, A. T., Steer, R. A., & Brown, G. K. (1996). *Beck depression inventory.* San Antonio: Psychological Corporation.

Benson, D. F. (1982). The treatable dementias. In D. F. Benson & D. Blumer (Eds.), *Psychiatric aspects of neurologic disease* (Vol. 2, pp. 123–148). New York: Grune & Stratton.

Benson, D. F. (1994). *The neurology of thinking.* New York: Oxford University Press.

Blumer, D., & Benson, D. F. (1975). Personality changes with frontal and temporal lobe lesions. In D. F. Benson & D. Blumer (Eds.), *Psychiatric aspects of neurologic disease* (Vol. 1, pp. 151–169). New York: Grune & Stratton.

Bryden, M. P., & Ley, R. G. (1983). Right-hemispheric involvement in the perception and expression of emotion in normal humans. In K. M. Heilman & P. Satz (Eds.), *Neuropsychology of human emotion* (pp. 6–44). New York: Guilford.

Butler, R. W., Rizzi, L. P., & Bandilla, E. B. (in press). The effects of childhood cancer treatment on two objective measures of psychological functioning. *Children's Health Care.*

Butler, R. W., & Satz, P. (1988). Individual psychotherapy with head-injured adults: Clinical notes for the practitioner. *Professional Psychology: Research and Practice, 19,* 536–541.

Caine, D. (1986). The neuropsychology of depression: The pseudodementia syndrome. In I. Grant & K. M. Adams (Eds.), *Neuropsychological assessment of neuropsychiatric disorders* (pp. 221–243). New York: Oxford University Press.

Cooper, I. S. (1976). *Living with chronic neurologic disease.* New York: W. W. Norton.

Fogel, B. S., & Sparadeo, F. R. (1985). Single case study: Focal cognitive deficits accentuated by depression. *Journal of Nervous and Mental Disease, 173,* 120–124.

Gualtieri, C. T., & Cox, D. R. (1991). The delayed neurobehavioral sequelae of traumatic brain injury. *Brain Injury, 5,* 219–232.

Gurdjian, E. S., & Gurdjian, E. S. (1976). Cerebral contusions: Reevaluation of the mechanism of their development. *Journal of Trauma, 16,* 35–51.

Harker, J. O., Satz, P., D'Elia, L. F., Miller, E. N., & Jin, S. (1997). Measuring depression in HIV-1 disease: A comparison of four instruments. Manuscript submitted for publication.

Heilman, K. M., Watson, R. T., & Bowers, D. (1983). Affective disorders associated with hemispheric disease. In K. M. Heilman & P. Satz (Eds.), *Neuropsychology of human emotion* (pp. 45–65). New York: Guilford.

Hibbard, M. R., Gordon, W. A., Egelko, S., & Langer, K. (1987). Issues in the diagnosis and cognitive therapy of depression in brain-damaged individuals. In A. Freeman & V. B. Greenwood (Eds.), *Cognitive therapy: Applications in psychiatric and medical settings* (pp. 183–198). New York: Human Sciences Press.

Jorge, R. E., Robinson, R. G., & Arndt, S. (1993). Are there symptoms that are specific for depressed mood in patients with traumatic brain injury. *Journal of Nervous and Mental Disease, 181,* 91–99.

Kinsella, G., Moran, C., Ford, B., & Ponsella, J. (1988). Emotional disorder and its assessment within the severe head injured population. *Psychological Medicine, 18,* 57–63.

Kovacs, M. (1992). *Children's depression inventory manual.* North Tonawanda, NY: Multi-Health Systems.

Kraus, M. F. (1995). Neuropsychiatric sequelae of stroke and traumatic brain injury: The role of psychostimulants. *International Journal of Psychiatry in Medicine, 25,* 39–51.

Lachar, D. (1984). *Multidimensional description of child personality: A manual for the personality inventory for children* (Rev.). Los Angeles, CA: Western Psychological Services.

Levin, H. S., Benton, A. L., & Grossman, R. G. (1982). *Neurobehavioral consequences of closed head injury.* New York: Oxford University Press.

Lewis, L., Athey, G. I., Eyman, J., & Saeks, S. (1992). Psychological treatment of adult psychiatric patients with traumatic frontal lobe injury. *Journal of Neuropsychiatry, 4,* 323–330.

Lezak, M. D. (1978). Living with the characterologically altered brain injured patient. *Journal of Clinical Psychiatry, 39,* 592–598.

Luria, A. R. (1980). *Higher cortical functions in man* (2nd ed., rev. & expanded). New York: Basic Books.

McKinlay, W. W., Brooks, D. N., Bond, M. R., Martinage, D. P., & Marshall, M. M. (1981). The short-term outcome of severe blunt head injury as reported by relatives of the injured persons. *Journal of Neurology, Neurosurgery & Psychiatry, 44,* 527–533.

Passler, M. A., Isaac, W., & Hynd, G. W. (1985). Neuropsychological development of behavior attributed to frontal lobe functioning in children. *Developmental Neuropsychology, 1,* 349.

Prigatano, G. P. (1987). Personality and psychosocial consequences after brain injury. In M. Meier, A. Benton, & L. Diller (Eds.), *Neuropsychological rehabilitation* (pp. 355–378). New York: Guilford.

Prigatano, G. P., & Schacter, D. L. (Eds.). (1991). *Awareness of deficit after brain injury.* New York: Oxford University Press.

Ross, E. (1981). The aprosodias. *Archives of Neurology, 38,* 561–569.

Robinson, R. G., & Price, T. R. (1982). Post-stroke depressive disorders: A follow-up study of 103 patients. *Stroke, 13,* 635–641.

Sackeim, H. A., Freeman, J., McElhiney, M., Coleman, E., Prudic, J., & Devanand, D. P. (1992). Effects of major depression on estimates of intelligence. *Journal of Clinical and Experimental Neuropsychology, 14,* 268–288.

Satz, P., Forney, D. L., Zaucha, K., Asarnow, R. F., Light, R., McCleary, C., Levin, H., Kelly, D., Bergsneider, M., Hovda, D., Martin, N., Namerow, N., & Becker, D. (in press). Depression, cognition, and functional correlates of recovery outcome after traumatic brain injury. *Brain Injury.*

Stark, K. D., Rouse, L. W., & Livingston, R. (1991). Treatment of depression during childhood and adolescence: Cognitive–behavioral procedures for the individual and family. In P. C. Kendall (Ed.), *Child and adolescent therapy* (pp. 165–206). New York: Guilford.

6.

Transference and Countertransference in Psychotherapy with Adults Having Traumatic Brain Injury

Lisa Lewis, Ph.D.

Leonard Diller (1994) notes that one of the trends in neuropsychological rehabilitation over the past 5 years has been a reemphasis of ego psychological constructs such as the self and self-efficacy as well as ego mechanisms of defense, including denial. He and others (Christensen, Henry, Ross, Kostasek, & Rosenthal, 1994) further note that primarily psychological factors such as strength of alliance formed with the rehabilitation team and degree of depression are better predictors of rehabilitation outcome than measures of neurological damage. It was over 50 years ago that Sir Charles Symonds (1937) said, "It is not only the kind of injury that matters but the kind of head" (p. 1087). So it is not that we are only now recognizing the role of psychological factors in determining the extent and rate of recovery following brain injury. It is only fairly recently, however, that we have begun to integrate an appreciation of psychological factors into our way of thinking and working.

We are aiming for an attitude in which the therapist and patient recognize the disability and deficits and also see more, see past them to the totality of the person and a vision of what that person might become. This implies an openness in the therapist to an empathic identification with the patient and an emotional reverberation with the patient's subjective experience. Out of this process frequently emerges an idealizing transference on the part of the patient to the therapist and a mirroring response from the therapist, processes described by Kohut (1977; Wolf, 1988) in general, and in particular by Klonoff and Lage (1991) in therapy with patients having traumatic brain injury. Some therapies never get to this point while others remain at this point until termination, but many evolve further. The Humpty Dumpty syndrome, true and complete restoration of the mind and self following brain injury, is the exception rather than the rule. Disillusionment and disappointment and working through of despair must also be a part of what we are open to experiencing with our patients (Lewis, Athey, Eyman, & Saeks, 1992)

Before talking about countertransference and transference in greater detail, it will be useful to briefly give an overview of the psychotherapy process so that transference and countertransference can be viewed in context (see Table 6.1). There

TABLE 6.1
Curative Factors in Psychotherapy

Technique		Relationship	
Education	*Real*	*Alliance*	*Transference & Countertransference*
Skills Training			
Clarification	Tx Frame	Hopefulness	
Confrontation	Respect	Shared goals	
Interpretation	Caring	Shared procedures	
Advice	Dependability		
Praise	Objective CT		

are two broad spheres of curative activity in psychotherapy. One sphere is the practical realm of therapeutic technique employed, such as education, skills training (e.g., relaxation, assertiveness, cognitive retraining), confrontation, clarification, interpretation, advice, praise, and so on. The other realm constitutes the intimate edge of the treatment relationship where existential meanings are discovered and created. The relationship consists of several components: The real relationship includes what Langs (1982) calls the treatment frame as well as the realistically expectable qualities of respect, caring, and dependability. The real relationship also includes what Ferenczi (1919) and Winnicott (1949) call the objective countertransference, meaning the kinds of responses the patient's behavior would elicit in nearly anyone. A second important ingredient of the therapeutic relationship is the alliance. The alliance is comprised of three factors: a sense of mutual trust and hopefulness in the effectiveness of treatment, an agreement on the problems and goals which will be the focus of therapy, and an agreement on the therapeutic techniques which will be employed. A last component of the therapeutic relationship, and one which will be the focus of the remainder of this chapter, is the transference and countertransference.

Transference and countertransference are ubiquitous. They happen not only in therapy but also in all relationships. They simply mean that current day relationships are perceived and experienced through the lens of our past significant relationships as they have affected our personality development. Our past is transferred or displaced onto our present. Depending upon how troubled our past relationships were and depending upon the extent to which we have individuated from our families of origin, transference and countertransference can be subtle and muted, a backdrop adding texture and nuance to our current relationships, or they can be in the foreground leading to maladaptive repetition of the same basic relational paradigms over and over again. In the latter case, transference and countertransference demand attention in the therapy process and can be powerful vehicles for change.

Transference and countertransference are two sides of the same coin. There are two models that are particularly helpful (see Table 6.2). They are simple enough to be remembered

TABLE 6.2
Transference and Countertransference

Racker:	Complementary: Feel as other person did
	Concordant: Feel what patient feels
Kohut:	Idealizing: Therapist as omnipotent, soothing presence
	Mirroring: Response validating self worth

and used during the nitty gritty of clinical hours and are also true to the clinical process. One model is formulated by Heinrich Racker (1968), an Argentinian analyst who trained with Melanie Klein and D. W. Winnicott. He speaks of complementary and concordant countertransference. In complementary countertransference, we feel what significant people in the patient's past, usually parents, felt in response to the patient's behavior. In concordant countertransference, we feel what the patient is feeling, or, perhaps more accurately, what the patient is defensively struggling not to feel. A second, and overlapping model, is provided by Kohut (1977). Nearly all patients, especially those who have experienced neuropsychological impairment, come to therapy with a large measure of narcissistic injury which needs to be addressed (Lewis & Rosenberg, 1990). Kohut describes the development of a self/object or idealizing transference in which the patient perceives the therapist as an omnipotent figure with whom the patient can merge and whose very presence is soothing and healing. The patient hungers for a mirroring response from the therapist, a confirming, validating response that Kohut likens to "the gleam in the mother's eye" and which provides the patient with a sense of self-worth.

An example will illustrate. Sarah, a 32-year-old single woman, sought treatment at Menninger 5 years after a significant traumatic brain injury (coma for 11 days, bilateral frontal lobe contusions, contusion of right temporal lobe, petechial cerebellar hemorrhage, brainstem contusion). Tragically, the injury was sustained in a car accident as Sarah was driving to visit her sister in the hospital who herself had been in a car accident 2 months before and rendered quadriplegic. Sarah had spent four of the last five years in medical hospitals and rehabilitation centers. In one rehabilitation center, she was befriended by her physical therapist who continued a social relationship with her after her discharge, eventually proposing marriage, which she accepted. The relationship was likely doomed from the start. Her fiancée was homosexual, he related to her more as if he were an omnipotent treater than a lover or friend, and he was financially dependent on her—she paid for everything out of the settlement from her accident. It seemed to be a Pygmalion sort of relationship where each of them tried to ignore the other's negative traits and transform the other into the person of their dreams. The negative traits could not be ignored and anger and resentment increasingly crept in.

At her concerned family's insistence, Sarah presented her fiancée with a prenuptial agreement designed to protect her finances. He did not sign it and two weeks later put her on a plane back to her mother. Her mother and father had divorced some 10 years ago. Sarah viewed her mother as a critical, demeaning, depressed woman who had been rejected by her father. She in turn idealized her father, a judge, whom she viewed as a knight in shining armor despite the fact that he was emotionally distant with her. After the breakup with her finacée, Sarah collapsed into deep, suicidal depression which failed to improve with outpatient psychotherapy and pharmacotherapy in her hometown. It was for this reason she came to Menninger.

In therapy with me, Sarah came to each session with written questions about herself, her life experiences, and her disorders, which included an ataxic gait, dysconjugate gaze, numerous cognitive deficits, and a preexisting narcissistic personality disorder with borderline features. She seemed to love to hear me talk, and the questions were designed to get me talking at length, to explain her to herself. For most of each session, she sobbed heavily about how badly life had treated her. Several times she told me I was the best, the very tip of the Ivory Tower, the best of the best. I found myself admiring her courage, her flashes of insight, her humor, and her pluck. Clearly, we had developed an idealizing and mirroring relationship. I also found myself quite taken with being the tip of the Ivory Tower. I suspected, and exploration with Sarah confirmed, that I was being idealized as her father was and financée had been, and that one of the bases of that idealization was splitting. She confirmed that she felt good about herself simply basking in the attention she got from me.

Predictably, the negative feelings being split off from our relationship began to intrude. I learned that Sarah was alienating a number of her peers and other staff by, for example, marching into a group session being led by her nurse and demanding immediate attention for her headache or telling patients in her group psychotherapy that she couldn't relate to their depression because no one had suffered anywhere near as much as she had. I found myself embarrassed by these reports and realized I was feeling a complementary countertransference of a parent for a child who went around the neighborhood acting entitled. I realized the danger of needing to change Sarah to make myself feel like a good therapist, and I suspected her mother had frequently felt the same way. In response to my question, Sarah indicated that she had indeed felt such expectations from her mother and often deliberately misbehaved to defeat her mother. Sarah began to act entitled with me; for example, insisting that I answer the same questions over and over or telling me, when I greeted her in the waiting room, "Pick that up, hon," referring to her backpack, and treating me like her servant. My embarrassment turned to irritation, again a complementary reaction I suspected I shared with her parents and fiancée. When I confronted her with how she irritated and demeaned others with her behavior she exploded, "How dare you!" and with hurt and angry glares laid into me for my inability to judge her in any way since I'd never had a head injury and I'd never suffered one tenth what she had.

It became clear to both of us that she waved the banner of her suffering proudly and was not going to give it up, despite her conscious wish to change. To her credit, she was able to reestablish an alliance and to explore the shift in her transference reaction to me. She recognized that by believing no one had suffered as she had she had reestablished her narcissistic equilibrium; now at last she was special, she was better than others. We came to call this her Queen for a Day complex. For those of you too young to remember, Queen for a Day was a TV program where women came on and told tales of woe to the audience who then applauded for the one who elicited the most sympathy. An applause meter was used to determine which woman had suffered the most and should be awarded a prize, such as a Maytag washer and dryer.

There then followed in the therapy with Sarah a very productive 4 months of therapy where the nuances of her narcissistic attachment to her injury and suffering were explored with all its ramifications. This led to a resolution of her depression, investment of her energy in pursuits more worthwhile than being Queen for a Day—such as getting her driver's license and entering vocational rehabilitation—an increase in her empathy with others, and significant improvement in her relationships with others.

In addition to illustrating complementary and concordant, idealizing and mirroring transference and countertransference reactions, the above case description also reveals a few

TABLE 6.3
Transference and Level of Ego Organization

Ego Strength:	A product of endowment, experience, neurological integrity
Ego functions:	Plan and execute action, regulate emotion and drive, reason, perceive, remember
Least Coherent:	Orbitofrontal Damage
Most Coherent:	Posterior Damage
Mediators:	Gender & Lifestage

additional important points (see Table 6.3). First, the intensity and coherence of the patient's transference is very much a product of their level of ego organization. Ego organization is in turn a product of experiential and developmental factors. It is also a product of neurological factors. A short list of primary autonomous ego functions described by Hartmann (1939/ 1958), Anna Freud (1936–1967), Rapaport, Gill, and Schafer (1968) and others, will sound familiar to the reader: planning and execution of purposeful behavior, regulation of emotion and drive, logical reasoning, perception, memory. These are neurologically mediated higher cognitive functions, especially executive functions associated principally with the frontal lobes. In clinical experience, it is patients who have had frontal lobe injury, especially orbitofrontal injury, who tend to have the most chaotically shifting transferences. Orbitofrontal injury is associated with disinhibition over lower brain regions, resulting in what John Hughlings Jackson (1931) termed regression or the emergence of positive symptoms. The resulting abrupt, reactive, and labile emergence of limbic emotion and drive can produce quickly shifting and intense transference states (Lewis, 1992). The content of the transference is in part determined by the individual's life experiences as they have shaped enduring character (e.g., dependent, erotic, aggressive transferences). Conversely, patients with posterior injury seem to have the least intense and most stable transferences.

Gender also influences transference reactions. Traumatic brain injuries are most commonly sustained by males in their late teens and early 20's. The injury occurs at a time when they need all of their resources to negotiate age-appropriate developmental tasks of forging and consolidating a cohesive adult identity. Complex themes of sexuality, emancipation from family of origin, selecting a life's work and mate must all be synthesized into an identity. The brain injury shatters this process and the patient regresses to an enforced state of dependence.

Usually it is the mother who takes the primary caretaking role (Solomon & Scherzer, 1991). She needs to function as an auxiliary ego-cortex for her adult son, exercising all of the protective and adaptive ego functions that have been diminished or lost due to brain dysfunction. Her son, often in a state of reduced self-awareness due to denial, impaired cognitive faculties for realistic self-appraisal, and/or anosognosia, can view her efforts as unwanted and unneeded intrusions. He resists her and goes his own way, only to encounter a crushing experience of failure or humiliation. He alternately clings and rebels, with neither position being adaptive. With a female therapist, as with the mother, these young men usually express a chaotic dependency attachment, alternately being clingy and then rebellious.

By way of additional illustration of the effects of gender and lesion locus on transference, two patients are both struggling with dependent transference longings. One is a 26-year-old man with diffuse but primarily bifrontal damage sustained in a motorcycle accident 7 years ago. He expresses his dependency by showing up at my office at any time, whether he has an appointment or not, but then often not keeping his scheduled appointments. During sessions, he alternately pleads for help and guidance then can be standoffish and haughty. Like many young men, he experienced his dependency longings with great ambivalence. Just as he was individuating and forming an adult male identity, the brain injury threw him back into a state of realistic dependence.

A second patient is a 52-year-old woman who sustained diffuse but primarily right parietal damage two years ago. She also struggled with dependent transference toward me but it was expressed in subtle ways of trying to make me happy and trying to make as few demands on me as possible, yet letting me know that she viewed me as a special person and the only one who could recreate a sense of wholeness and meaning in her life. Thus, in ways we are beginning to learn about, lesion locus, gender, and dynamic conflict interact to alter the form and content of transference reactions.

The case of Sarah also illustrates that we as therapists can have countertransference to multiple aspects of the patient and that countertransferences of opposite emotional valence can coexist or succeed one another (Laatsch, Rothke, & Burke, 1993; see Figure 6.1) Our perception of the patient's deficits can elicit countertransference. Typical reactions include a view of the patient as someone who has been cruelly and unfairly damaged, evoking great sympathy within us and an intense longing to restore them to wholeness. Conversely, we can feel overwhelmed by the enormity of their suffering and need, leading us to withdraw (Ball, 1988; Lewis, 1991). Second, countertransference can be elicited by how the patient perceives his or her own deficits. A patient's denial of deficit or a patient's sense that the injury entitles them to special treatment, or a patient's magnification of deficit, all can elicit varied countertransference reactions, depending on the therapist, but typically elicit irritation and anger (Langer, 1994). The countertransference anger can then find expression in overly zealous confrontation of the patient's perception of deficit. At times, the anger can be defended against, leading the therapist to collude with the patient's misperception of deficit.

Last, the patient's transference toward us can elicit countertransference. Just as the content of the patient's transference is determined by their unique conflicts and characters, so too are therapists' countertransference reactions. In response to being idealized, most therapists feel pride and an increased

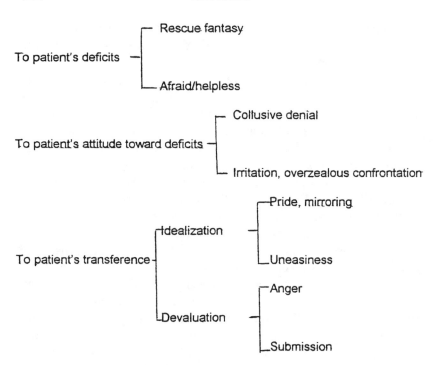

Figure 6.1 Countertransference

sense of liking and warmth for the patient. At other times or for other therapists, being idealized elicits uneasiness and increased distance. Being placed on a pedestal can leave the therapists uneasy about there being nowhere to go but down, and uneasy about the inevitable disappointment to come when the illusion of perfection is not sustained. In response to being devalued (ignored, deskilled, belittled, competed with), most therapists feel anger. However, others, either fearful of confrontation-conflict or as a result of employing reaction formation against their anger, can become submissive or overly conciliatory in the face of devaluation. Though it may feel more comfortable to be the very tip of the Ivory Tower than to be relegated to the role of applauder in the audience of Queen for a Day, both countertransference reactions can be explored with benefit to the patient. The goal for the therapist is to recognize, reflect on, and understand the meanings of countertransference so as to foster insight in the patient.

While it is commonly accepted that transference and countertransference can be vehicles of change when recognized and understood, the process of attaining insight is not formulaic. As Gunther (1994) states, the price an effective team pays for significant therapeutic involvement with patients having severe brain damage is periodic subjective distress and less than optimal professional functioning. The solutions he cites are to better understand the patient's subjective experience, have a firm grounding in the essentials of modern psychoanalytically based depth psychology, attain awareness of one's inner world acquired through self-reflection and psychoanalysis, and schedule regular and candid staff meetings with a consultant. The gain is that by listening more fully to ourselves, we learn what is going on in the minds of our patients.

Pepping (1993) provides a number of helpful suggestions about how to make productive use of transference and countertransference. A psychoeducational approach to teaching patients about transference, especially self-defeating or masochistic styles of relating, can be taken. For example, patients can be given the mnemonic of the 3 Ps: pick, provoke, perceive. That is, patients can be helped to understand that conflictual and painful ways of relating, forged in childhood, can lead them to find someone who will mistreat them (pick), aggravate someone into treating them unfairly (provoke), or distort their view of reality into seeing themselves as injured by others to a greater degree than is actually true (perceive). Then, when events in treatment or daily life contain strong transferential elements, the patient can be reminded of this mnemonic as encouragement to reflect on the meaning of the maladaptive interchange.

Often, when a therapist is trying to help a patient recognize and reflect on transference, the patient's anxiety increases with a proportional increase in defensiveness. A strong dose of support can be helpful in decreasing anxiety and sustaining that alliance. Pepping (1993) refers to this as the sandwich technique. Confrontation (the act of drawing the patient's attention to the transference behaviors) and interpretation (offering a way of understanding the meaning of the behavior) are preceded and followed by praise for accomplishments made, positive traits and talents, and for persevering with the hard work of treatment.

In addition to the sandwich technique, Pine's (1986) suggestion of "striking when the iron is cold" is useful. This is a way of doing expressive work in a supportive fashion. One waits until the patient has recovered his or her composure before embarking on efforts at reflection and insight. In other words, interpretations are made deliberately late, after the moment of emotional intensity has past and the patient can think more clearly and with some appropriate distance.

The work with the countertransference follows the same general principles of awareness (confrontation) and insight (interpretation). The therapist sorts out the part of the countertransference having to do with his or her own issues from those having to do with the patient's inner world. The latter is then introduced into the work as either a confrontation or interpretation. For example, the therapist, based on his or her own countertransference anger, might say, "I wonder if you have been feeling some anger towards me" (confrontation), or "I wonder whether your irritability towards me has to do with feeling I expect too much of you" (complimentary countertransference), or "Perhaps you are being irritable with me as a way of making me feel the anger you have felt over your situation" (concordant countertransference).

CONCLUSION

To sum up, as in psychotherapy with neurologically intact individuals, transference and countertransference in psychotherapy with adults having brain injury or stroke are potentially powerful vehicles for change as well as powerful sources of resistance. The form of a patient's transference, its coherence and intensity, is determined by structural factors, primarily the level of ego organization. Level of ego organization is the product of constitutional endowment, character, and locus and extent of neurological injury. The content of the transference, especially its dynamic themes, is determined by historical and current life experiences, including the phenomenology and psychological meaning of being brain injured. The patient's experience and expression of being impaired in turn elicits countertransference in the therapist, with gender playing a prominent mediating role.

Karl Menninger (1958) said that the countertransference is dangerous only when it is forgotten about. One of the values of working with an interdisciplinary team in a milieu oriented program is that the potential for recognizing and therapeutically processing transference and countertransference reactions is multiplied (Prigatano, 1989, 1994). When working as a solo psychotherapist, it is very useful for the therapist to have adequate time to reflect on sessions so as to be able to recognize countertransference and engage in self-analysis to learn what it means for the self and the patient. Yet, as Freud said, the problem with self-analysis *is* the countertransference. In some instances of stalemates, the opportunity to consult with a colleague or to seek focused therapy of our own can be invaluable.

REFERENCES

Ball, J. D. (1988) Psychotherapy with head injured patients. *Medical Psychotherapy, 1,* 15–22.

Christensen, B. K., Henry, R. R., Ross, T. P., Kostasek, R. S., & Rosenthal, M. (1994). The role of depression in rehabilitation outcome during acute recovery from traumatic brain injury. *Advances in Medical Psychotherapy, 7,* 27–38.

Diller, L. (1994). Finding the right treatment combinations: Changes in rehabilitation over the past five years. In A-L Christensen & B. P. Uzell (Eds.), *Brain injury and neuropsychological rehabilitation. International perspectives* (pp. 1–16). Hillsdale, NJ: Lawrence Erlbaum.

Ferenczi, S. (1919). On the technique of psychoanalysis. In *Further contributions to the theory and technique of psychoanalysis* (pp. 177–188). London: Hogarth Press, 1950.

Freud, A. (1967). *The ego and mechanisms of defense.* New York: International Universities Press. (Original work published 1936.)

Gunther, M. S. (1994). Countertransference issues in staff caregivers who work to rehabilitate catastrophic-injury survivors. *American Journal of Psychotherapy, 48,* 208–220.

Hartmann, H. (1958). *Ego psychology and the problem of adaptation.* New York: International Universities Press. (Original work published 1939.)

Jackson, J. Hughlings (1931). *Selected writings of John Hughlings Jackson* (Vols. 1 & 2). London: Hodder & Stoughton.

Klonoff, P. S., & Lage, G. A. (1991). Narcissistic injury in patients with traumatic brain injury. *Journal of Head Trauma Rehabilitation, 6,* 11–21.

Kohut, H. (1977). *The restoration of the self.* New York: International Universities Press.

Laatsch, L., Rothke, S., & Burke, W. F. (1993). Countertransference and the multiple amputee patient: Pitfalls and opportunities in rehabilitation medicine. *Archives of Physical Medicine and Rehabilitation, 74,* 644–648.

Langer, K. G. (1994). Depression and denial in psychotherapy of persons with disabilities. *American Journal of Psychotherapy, 48,* 181–194.

Langs, R. (1982). *Psychotherapy, a basic text.* New York: Jason Aronson.

Lewis, L. (1991). A framework for developing a psychotherapy treatment plan with brain-injured patients. *Journal of Head Trauma Rehabilitation, 6,* 22–29.

Lewis, L. (1992). Two neuropsychological models and their psychotherapeutic implications. *Bulletin of the Menninger Clinic, 56,* 20–32.

Lewis, L., Athey, G. I., Eyman, J., & Saeks, S. (1992). Psychological treatment of adult psychiatric patients with traumatic frontal lobe injury. *Journal of Neuropsychiatry, 4,* 323–330.

Lewis, L., & Rosenberg, S. J. (1990). Psychoanalytic psychotherapy with brain-injured adult psychiatric patients. *Journal of Nervous and Mental Disease, 178,* 69–77.

Menninger, K. (1958). *Theory of psychoanalytic technique.* New York: Basic Books.

Pepping, M. (1993). Transference and countertransference issues in brain injury rehabilitation: Implications for staff training. In C. J. Durgin, N. D. Schmidt, & L. J. Fryer (Eds.), *Staff development and clinical intervention in brain injury rehabilitation* (pp. 87–104). Gaithersburg, MD: Aspen.

Pine, F. (1986). Supportive psychotherapy. A psychoanalytic perspective. *Psychiatric Annals, 16,* 515–529.

Prigatano, G. P. (1989). Bring it up in the milieu: Toward effective traumatic brain injury rehabilitation interaction. *Rehabilitation Psychology, 34,* 135–144.

Prigatano, G. P. (1994). Individuality, lesion location, and psycho-
    therapy after brain injury. In A. L. Christensen & B. P. Uzzell
    (Eds.), *Brain injury and neuropsychological rehabilitation. Interna-
    tional perspectives.* Hillsdale, NJ: Lawrence Erlbaum.
Racker, H. (1968). *Transference and countertransference.* New York:
    International Universities Press.
Rapaport, D., Gill, M. M., & Schafer, R. (1968). *Diagnostic psychological
    testing.* New York: International Universities Press.
Solomon, C. R., & Scherzer, B. P. (1991). Some guidelines for family
    therapists working with the traumatically brain injured and their
    families. *Brain Injury, 5,* 253–266.
Symonds, C. P. (1937). Mental disorder following head injury. *Pro-
    ceedings of the Royal Society of Medicine, 30,* 1081–1094.
Winnicott, D. W. (1949). Hate in the countertransference. *Interna-
    tional Journal of Psycho-Analysis, 30,* 69–75.
Wolf, E.S. (1988). *Treating the self-elements of clinical self psychology.*
    New York: Guilford.

PART III

Interplay of Psychotherapy and Cognitive Remediation in Individual Treatment

7.

Application of Cognitive Rehabilitation Techniques in Psychotherapy

Linda Laatsch, Ph.D.

INTRODUCTION

The central goal of psychotherapy is to effect a beneficial change in a client through verbal or symbolic interaction (Langer, 1992). To do this, therapists frequently ask their clients to reflect on their current emotional experiences, discuss long-standing conflicts, and expand on their knowledge about themselves. Unfortunately, common consequences following brain dysfunction include significant cognitive impairments such as memory deficits, limited concentration, impaired perception and communication, and difficulties with reading, writing, math, planning, self-awareness, and judgment (National Head Injury Foundation, 1989). These impairments can have a significant impact on the client's ability to communicate needs and conflicts in therapy, effectively perceive their own and other's emotional state, and reliably recall therapeutic interventions during and after therapy.

For almost 40 years, cognitive deficits following a brain dysfunction have been treated with what can now be identified as cognitive rehabilitation therapy (CRT). Cognitive rehabilitation therapy is broadly defined as those activities that improve a patient with brain injury's "higher cerebral functioning or help the patient to better understand the nature of those difficulties while teaching him or her methods of compensation" (Klonoff, O'Brien, Prigatano, Chiapello, & Cunningham, 1989, p. 37). Experts frequently comment on the rapid growth of cognitive rehabilitation as a treatment modality in the past 15 years (Gianutsos, 1991; Lehr, 1990). Parents and loved ones of individuals with brain dysfunction are demanding cognitive rehabilitation services. Therefore, most brain dysfunction facilities offer cognitive rehabilitation as part of their treatment. Mazmanian and collaborators (Mazmanian, Martin, & Kreutzer, 1991) in their comprehensive survey found that 91% of "brain injury programs" offered in-house cognitive rehabilitation. Bach-y-Rita (1992), well known in the field of brain rehabilitation, stated, although following brain dysfunction there is generally some early recovery, specific rehabilitation programs are usually required to obtain later gains. He also stated that "if recovery is not expected or strived for with active participation of the disabled person, little recovery is obtained" (Matthews, Harley, & Malec, 1987, p. 191). Systematic studies of individuals 5 to 7 years post brain damage have revealed that without treatment many individuals do not continue to progress and may even get worse (Gianutsos, 1991).

The recent rapid growth of the field of CRT has lead to the development of a variety of models of cognitive rehabilitation and a variety of names for the many types of treatment. Popular names include neuropsychological rehabilitation, cognitive retraining, behavioral rehabilitation, and cognitive remediation. In addition, related therapeutic approaches that focus on a specific cognitive problem include memory rehabilitation and perceptual rehabilitation. Currently, there is uncertainty in defining extent of cognitive rehabilitation therapy as a result, professional standards are currently being developed (Mazmanian et al., 1991), and guidelines for the field have been published (Matthews et al., 1987).

As defined broadly above, CRT is very similar to a definition of psychotherapy. Both techniques involve facilitation of change and both involve interventions that impact the emotional and cognitive status of the client receiving treatment.

Stern, a psychiatrist providing guidelines for psychotherapy with the neuropsychologically impaired, states that psychotherapy is designed "to 'assist' nature in arriving at higher functional levels by integrating the components of the various clinical syndromes" (Stern, 1985, p. 84).

Within the last 10 years numerous papers have been written describing psychotherapy with individuals who have neuropsychological impairments (Cicerone, 1989; Langer, 1992; Langer & Padrone, 1992; Lewis, 1992; Lewis, Athey, Eyman, & Saeks, 1992; Morris & Bleiberg, 1986; Prigatano & Klonoff, 1988; Laatsch, 1996). Application of standard theoretical psychotherapeutic approaches are described, and the impact of the neuropsychological deficits on the therapeutic process are described in detail. Individuals with neuropsychological impairments frequently exhibit lack of insight, decreased awareness of their current abilities and deficits, and a general loss of their sense of self (Prigatano, 1995). Cicerone (1989) also suggests that rigidity and defensiveness may also hinder a client's ability to benefit from psychotherapeutic interventions. Neuropsychologically impaired clients may focus on the "old self" (whom they were before their injury) and almost perseverate on things they recall from the past and who they might have become without the injury. Since some or even all of these factors may influence a client's self-awareness and mental flexibility, psychotherapists may find it difficult to develop and sustain an effective therapeutic relationship with a client who has neuropsychological deficits.

Even though neuropsychological impairments can hinder the client's ability to make therapeutic changes in their emotional status, some clients, as a result of their trauma, are more open to change than they were prior to their injury. The trauma and the realization of previous health-threatening behaviors, may provide for some clients an opportunity for reevaluation. All clients who have experienced a brain dysfunction need to "establish meaning in their life in the face of (not despite) their impairments" (Prigatano, 1995, p. 87). Some brain injured individuals stop abusing drugs and alcohol thereby having a beneficial effect on their life-style. Clients will generally seek to answer a question concerning, "Why did this happen to me?" (Prigatano, 1995, p. 88). A change in how the client views his life and how he defines his priorities may result. Therefore, although psychotherapists working with individuals who have experienced a brain dysfunction may be faced with many obstacles in therapy, some clients may be more ready for change because of the trauma they have experienced.

UTILIZATION OF CRT TECHNIQUES IN PSYCHOTHERAPY WITH CLIENTS WHO HAVE NEUROPSYCHOLOGICAL IMPAIRMENTS

There are many reasons why the integration of cognitive rehabilitation techniques into a psychotherapy environment with brain injured clients would assist treatment. The integration of treatment is natural, a detailed examination of psychotherapy with neuropsychologically impaired clients reveals that many CRT techniques are embedded in psychotherapy. For example, if at the end of the therapy session, important topics are reviewed for the client, the therapist has facilitated rehearsal of material and assisted in encoding. In addition, the integration is supported by extensive research that has demonstrated the effectiveness of CRT with brain injured clients. Gianutsos (1991) feels that, given the current research describing the efficacy of CRT following brain dysfunction, a no-treatment group is not ethical. Very recently, CRT was related to significant changes in SPECT imaging (Single Photon Emission Computed Tomography) in a longitudinal study with patients with diverse brain injuries. A significant increase in blood flow redistribution was seen in areas adjacent to the brain dysfunction and also in areas of the brain associated with the specific CRT strategies utilized. It is theorized that CRT serves to "turn on plasticity" even in patients many years post brain dysfunction (Laatsch, 1996; Laatsch, Jobe, Synchra, Lin, & Blend, 1997). Since there is much research suggesting the effectiveness of CRT, it is expected that the use of CRT techniques would most likely serve to enhance the psychotherapeutic endeavor.

Finally, because of the similarity of the treatment techniques and goals, the inclusion of CRT techniques can only serve to facilitate treatment effectiveness. The level of integration of CRT techniques into the psychotherapeutic session can be varied according to specific patient needs and goals. Below, three levels of integration of CRT techniques, casual, moderate, and an alternating approach, are described. Examples of each specific technique are described at each level and client illustrations have been provided to facilitate understanding of each of the specific applications. This chapter does not attempt to describe the broad range of CRT techniques available, but instead how some CRT techniques can be easily integrated into psychotherapy with neuropsychologically impaired clients. CRT techniques are described in detail in recent issues of the *Journal of Cognitive Rehabilitation* and in many books, such as Parente and Herrmann (1996).

CASUAL INTEGRATION OF CRT TECHNIQUES IN PSYCHOTHERAPY

A casual or occasional integration of CRT techniques into psychotherapy with neuropsychologically impaired clients will depend on the specific neuropsychological and emotional limitations of the client. As is true in psychotherapy, the client will have to be open to application of the techniques and be able to trust their therapist sufficiently to believe that the technique might be effective. A central goal in CRT is to facilitate the client's ability to think about their own thinking. This technique is very familiar to educators and is defined by educators as "metacognition." The use of SPECT in CRT cases has demonstrated that effective CRT, which results in neuropsychological improvements and the successful return to a functional occupation or school, generally involves a significant increase in resting blood flow in the frontal and prefrontal regions of the brain (Laatsch et al., 1997). Self-awareness, initiation, and motivation are known to be mediated by these areas of the brain. Therefore, even the casual introduction of CRT techniques should include an effort to involve the client's thinking about their own cognitive limitations and effective compensation strategies. Casual introduction of CRT techniques will be described for individuals with neuropsychological impairments in attention and memory, communication, and executive processing.

Deficits in attention and memory are known to be one of the most common neuropsychological deficits following brain dysfunction. Although clients with severe memory deficits sometimes are unable to remember that they have a memory problem, many clients with mild to moderate memory difficulties are aware of their memory problems. Since getting the client to the therapy session is the first essential step in promoting therapeutic changes, all clients need a mechanism that will allow this to regularly occur. Clients who do not use an appointment or date book should be provided with one (even Freud, on occasion, is known to have provided his psychoanalytic clients with food!). A date book facilitates organization and provides a mechanism for rehearsal. Most clients respond well to the use of a date book which can facilitate pride and independence. In addition to recording the next scheduled appointment, clients can be taught to use it to maintain their own medication schedule. One client who was completely dependent on his spouse for his medication schedule was taught to list the times he took his medication on each day in the date book and cross that time off once he took his medication. This client was taught to have his date book open on the kitchen table and learned to use the book continuously. This client, who was also being seen in couple therapy, revealed that the simple use of the date book helped to restore a more independent relationship with his wife.

A date book, with enough space, can be used to provide a way for the client to practice therapeutic techniques promoted in therapy. Therapeutic goals can be written in the date book at the end of each session. A client who needs to practice relaxation techniques prior to the next session but states that he or she "forgot to do it" can be provided with reminders in their date book. In addition, the client can use it to record the use of therapeutic techniques outside of therapy.

Patients with memory disorders will need numerous repetitions during sessions to help recall suggestions and goals in therapy. Visual elaboration or simple rehearsal of the suggestion will usually assist recall. Symbolism, as described by Lewis and Langer (1994), especially if utilizing a visual image, can provide the visual stimuli needed to assist recall. For example, a patient with a storage deficit (unable to regularly store new information for effective recall) was provided with the image "in one ear and out the other." This image was used repeatedly in therapy sessions to assist the client's recall of her neuropsychological impairments and increase her self-awareness. Although it is most beneficial if clients are able to spontaneously develop their own "symbol" to illustrate a concept, clients with communication or initiation deficits might need to be supplied with a symbol to illustrate a concept.

It is well known by neuropsychologists that communication deficits can result from damage to both left and right cerebral hemispheres. Communication deficits resulting from damage from the dominant hemisphere (usually left hemisphere) are generally more obvious and may involve both receptive and expressive language skills. Many clients following brain dysfunction have difficulty with double negatives or statements which involve inverted commands, such as "before pressing the letter 'Q' press the letter 'M' " (Bracy, 1994). Unfortunately, abstract speech patterns are frequent in therapy sessions because the issues being addressed are often complex. Therapeutic approaches may be ineffective because the client did not understand the complexities of the communication. Clients with communication deficits will need to be asked to restate the issue in their own words. Clients can be asked to "tell me what we have talked about" or asked to recall what they were going to work on prior to the next session.

Clients with communication deficits that involve expression might benefit from rehabilitation techniques typically employed in speech therapy. When the therapist is able to assist in word-finding by suggesting alternate choices or providing an initial sound, the client's sense of trust and connection with their therapist is reaffirmed. Just as speech therapists utilize exaggerated speech to assist in articulation deficits, a client with expressive speech deficits can be asked to use exaggerated emotional expression to facilitate communication. Again, to facilitate self-awareness, the client should be made aware that a specific approach is being used because of existing neuropsychological deficits. The use of techniques designed to facilitate communication should be promoted at home and modeled for family members if possible. The use of exaggeration or modeling helps to facilitate immediate communication with a client, but these techniques are also compensation techniques that can be taught to assist communication outside the therapeutic environment.

Clients who have extensive executive processing deficits, such as difficulties in motivation, insight, problem solving, and initiation, generally require the most creativity and patience on the part of the therapist. A client, 20 years post severe brain dysfunction that required the removal of his right frontal lobe, began every session for 2 months with the statement, "If I had a gun I'd shoot myself." After checking carefully for suicidal ideation, it was determined that this statement was part of a perservative thought pattern that involved a focus on his past self and who he "could have become." There was a sense that this patient found himself "stuck" in a depressive cycle of thoughts and was calling for help in restructuring his thinking about himself. As needed with patients who have deficits in executive processing, a directive, cognitive behavioral approach was taken. This client developed self-statements, called "behavior resolutions," such as, "I am the most important part of my recovery and I will think about the here-and-now." These statements were written by the client in his daily recorder and repeated every evening. He was made aware that he was "stuck" on thoughts about how "bad" his life is, and an attempt was made to break the cycle with new self-statements. The depressive, suicidal thoughts were found to quickly decease using this technique.

Clients with impulsivity, impaired insight, and poor self-control in therapy can be asked to establish a contract, signed by both client and therapist, to define appropriate behavior in therapy. The rules listed in the contract (such as, "I will not ask my therapist personal questions") need to be closely followed by both client and therapist to facilitate self-control. It is hoped that the "rules" would be internalized so that, following excessive practice and modeling, the client would be able to use the established rules to guide behavior outside therapy, such as on a job interview. Occasional or casual use of CRT techniques, which include facilitation of self-awareness through modeling of correct behavior and the establishment of rules to guide behavior, helps the client to compensate for existing neuropsychological deficits.

MODERATE INTEGRATION OF CRT TECHNIQUES

Moderate application of CRT techniques is loosely defined as application of CRT as part of every therapy session. It can provide a challenging but safe, artificial environment for both patient and therapist. It provides a vehicle for increasing the therapist's understanding of the patient's cognitive and emotional state by providing examples of current functioning and behavior. The psychotherapist too can benefit in numerous ways when CRT is integrated into every therapy session. On a basic level, with clients unable to describe or recall details of daily activities, cognitive rehabilitation tasks serve to provide concrete examples of behavior such as the client's ability to cope with challenges or frustrations. Because the behavior occurs during the session, it is readily available for discussion between client and psychotherapist. Furthermore, cognitive rehabilitation therapy can reveal subtle cognitive changes in a client's neuropsychological functioning that may imply that a change in psychotherapeutic focus is now possible. Finally, since there is a similarity in themes addressed in cognitive rehabilitation and psychotherapy, joint treatment can serve to enhance progress in treatment. For example, both CRT and psychotherapy require the client to think about their own internal state, cognitive and emotional, and thereby facilitate self-awareness.

Assisting the client with brain dysfunction to use a date book or appointment calendar at the beginning of therapy, and instructing the client to bring the date book in for every session, provides a connection with the client's outside world.

Because of their brain dysfunction, clients are often unable to recall details of recent significant events. Clients can be instructed to use the date book to record significant events occurring each day (a date book with sufficient room for daily recording is essential here). One client who was shot through the left side of his head and sustained extensive damage in both frontal lobes, was asked to write daily sentences in his date book describing one thing he did independently. He was able to write a unique sentence every day but, within each sentence, verbal perservation was evident. In reviewing the date book in session, it was possible to talk about his achievements like, "How was it to make your own sandwich for lunch?" Looking at the date book at the beginning of each session provides topics for discussion and allows for the exploration significant relationships and events. The date book can be used as a diary to record emotions or difficult situations faced by clients, and it can be used to record achievement. The date book can also be used for homework assignments. A date book/appointment calendar is typically called an "external memory device" by CRT specialists but also can function as a therapeutic aide in psychotherapy.

When CRT is included in each therapy session the clinician needs to decide how and when to include CRT in the sessions. For some clients it is important to address emotional issues early in the session. The emotional needs may hinder the client's ability to work on their cognitive impairments in CRT. If the cognitive tasks used to illustrate current cognitive status and develop compensation strategies are standardized and scores are regularly recorded (such as done on computerized cognitive rehabilitation tasks), the impact of emotional issues can often be seen. Therefore it might be necessary to return to overriding emotional issues after attempting CRT. Alternately, some clients, especially those with reduced self-awareness, can benefit from CRT in the first part of the session, rather than the final part of the session. This is illustrated in the following case.

A highly educated, young professional woman who developed anoxic encephalitis following an asthma attack that resulted in a respiratory arrest, was found to have great difficulties expressing her emotions except in a very superficial manner. She tended to prefer to minimize her emotional response to her losses and drastic changes in her life. Providing both CRT and psychotherapy in her sessions was thought to facilitate her ability to understand the impact of her deficits in everyday life. The cognitive rehabilitation tasks selected at this point in her recovery revealed that the client tended to focus and perseverate on inessential details rather than develop an effective overall plan in simple problem-solving tasks. Following CRT addressing this difficulty, this client reported, laughing, that she had learned that her professional license had been used to bill for treatment that she could no longer perform following her brain dysfunction. When her unusual emotional reaction was explored further it was striking that she was unable to identify the serious implications of the use of her license by other professionals. She was focused on, "I've been working so hard to go back to work again and here I've been 'working' and I didn't know it." The insight she was able to derive from the situation was limited to an immediate, personal implication, but she was unable to express an understanding of the larger implications of the situation. Her performance on the cognitive rehabilitation tasks was used to help her understand her difficulties in conceptualizing the larger implications of the situation. Just as she was unable to see the forest for the trees on the problem-solving tasks earlier in the session, she could not identify the larger implications of the situation. The use of CRT and psychotherapy in the same session also allowed the therapist to develop more insight into how the client's current cognitive impairments might impact her understanding of incidents that occurred in her everyday life.

Including CRT in sessions with clients who have neuropsychological deficits can be uncomfortable for both client and therapist. Therapists early in their training in cognitive rehabilitation may find themselves more comfortable with "talk" therapy and find themselves tending to emphasize psychotherapy in sessions. One student, in his second CRT session, asked his supervisor if he could just do psychotherapy with the client he was assigned because "she needs that too." He was able to demonstrate good insight into his own reaction. He could identify that watching the client struggle with the cognitive rehabilitation tasks made him feel uncomfortable, and therefore, because of his discomfort, he felt he would prefer to do only psychotherapy.

In a well-designed cognitive rehabilitation program, the specific neuropsychological deficits of the clients are identified and emphasized and therefore the client is often made acutely aware of his or her limitations. This can be minimized by careful selection of cognitive rehabilitation activities and the use of a developmental model of CRT (Bolger, 1980; Christensen, 1987; Laatsch, 1983). In this approach, cognitive rehabilitation tasks designed to improve attention, processing speed, and concentration are presented before tasks involving higher cognitive operations (such as memory and visual perception). While problem-solving skills are addressed in the final stages of CRT, throughout the therapy there is an emphasis on the patient's ability to think about their own thinking (metacognition).

Moderate integration of CRT into individual sessions with clients requires flexibility. There is a need to integrate the treatment in a way that is most beneficial for the client given his or her current cognitive and emotional status. Clients in treatment right after the acute phase of brain dysfunction experience relatively rapid changes, and therefore the client's cognitive and emotional needs will most likely change during treatment. Although early in treatment a client may benefit from beginning each therapy session with CRT, later in treatment the same client might require that the therapist begin the session with psychotherapy. An increased self-awareness and a prevalence of emotional issues often occurs as treatment progresses. The client described above with anoxic encephalitis was able to benefit from 3 months of psychotherapy following discharge from CRT because, as her insight increased, she experienced periodic depressions related to her difficulty obtaining employment within her vocation.

ALTERNATING CRT AND PSYCHOTHERAPY

For some clients it may be helpful to overtly structure the treatment by alternating between CRT sessions and psychotherapy sessions. This is only effective if the client can meet for treatment more than one time per week. In these cases, the patient should be informed that the focus of sessions will be alternated and that reminders be provided, "Today we will do cognitive rehabilitation." A different area of the treatment room might be selected for each type of treatment. In this way, the physical setting will be a reminder of the type of treatment scheduled. If the same therapist participates in each treatment, the CRT can provide an opportunity to observe the patient's ability to tolerate a limited amount of frustration and the patient's ability to self-evaluate current abilities. Again, observation of the client while doing CRT provides insight into what it might be like for the client to be challenged by his environment (such as on a job or at home) given his or her current status. This insight can be utilized in the next psychotherapy session scheduled and helps the psychotherapist develop more empathy for the client's emotional struggles.

A client who had a motor vehicle accident that resulted in a diffuse brain dysfunction began alternating CRT-psychotherapy treatment 9 months after his brain injury. During the initial interview he expressed frustration that he was still "having trouble going to college" and that he wanted to complete college so that he could train to be a commercial airline pilot. Initial CRT sessions revealed that this client tended to focus on and become very frustrated with the errors he made during the tasks. Even when performance was adequate, he would frequently be unable to continue the task following a minor error. Further exploration revealed that this individual had maintained unrealistic high expectations that hindered both his ability to work effectively with his existing mild deficits and to use compensation strategies when needed. The psychotherapy allowed this client to express his prior beliefs about being "all-powerful," perfect, and infallible, and slowly helped him incorporate knowledge about his new self. As he continued to work on the cognitive rehabilitation tasks, overt frustration diminished as the patient began to employ effective strategies to the presented tasks. At the conclusion of treatment, this client entered the Air Force hoping to become involved in airplane maintenance.

If the same therapist alternates CRT and psychotherapy in treatment he or she has the benefit of detailed knowledge about both the client's current emotional struggles and cognitive abilities. This can serve to facilitate integration of treatment and allow for the transfer of cognitive strategies to assist emotional adjustment. Conceptually, the therapist who integrates both types of treatment is helping the client separate "soul" from "mind." The therapist also provides guidance in the integration of the two components of self in the most beneficial way.

SUMMARY

Integrating CRT into psychotherapy with neuropsychologically impaired clients can be accomplished many ways; three techniques are suggested in this chapter. The benefits of integrating treatment are thought to be substantial but unfortunately there are disadvantages associated with this type of treatment. First, the treatment personnel need to have specific and well-developed clinical skills. The emotional investment that the therapist needs to be able to make at least doubles when both types of treatment are done by one therapist. Although the therapist can certainly improve his or her empathic stance through the painful reminders provided by the cognitive tasks, the activities may also be an uncomfortable reminder of the vulnerable nature of human existence and the significant impact that cognitive deficits have on everyday living. The therapist needs to effectively process and understand his or her countertransference response to the increased intensity of the relationship. The client, in turn, may become more dependent on the therapist because of the comprehensive nature of joint CRT–psychotherapy treatment.

It is felt that the benefit of combining CRT and psychotherapy is substantial. From the client's point of view, there is often no clear distinction between the cognitive and emotional dimensions. This is clearly and beautifully described by Rob Taylor in "From the Patient's Point of View" (Taylor, 1996). He describes his loss as a "fierce severance, as of sword, came the cognitive leaving of my accumulated world" while his emotional response is described as "despairing months of deepening frustration." The poem describes the joy of getting help from an individual with "keys to all the locks" (see p. 146).

Integrated treatment, including both CRT and psychotherapy, can facilitate change because a deeper, more personal approach is taken with the client. The similarity between the intentions of both CRT and psychotherapy suggests that integrating the two treatments is quite possible. Typically, a therapist needs to act as an auxiliary ego in supportive psychotherapy (Lewis & Rosenberg, 1990). In treatment with neuropsychologically impaired clients the therapist must also act as an auxiliary "cortex," helping the client structure and learn to compensate for cognitive limitations (Lewis & Rosenberg, 1990). It is believed that by incorporating CRT techniques, the therapist's ability to empathize with the client is enhanced and thereby facilitating change in clients with neuropsychological impairments.

APPENDIX A

Walking Tall

As quickly as a blink of eye,
Fierce severance, as of sword,
Came the cognitive leaving of
My accumulated world.
Comprehending that disaster,
It's scope, it's devastation,
Settled slowly, through despairing months
Of deepening frustration.
The curtain fell; sickly gray, not black,
The fog of living while not here.
The world alleged I wasn't me.
I denied, in total fear.
I longed to be where "I" had gone,
Could not discern the way.
Unable to perceive my plight,
Depression deepened every day.
Since I could not go to me
Soon I'd return again!
That surely thus it had to be
I clung to through the pain!
Enveloped in the blanket of
Despair and weary fight,
While losing all, so futilely . . .
Suddenly appeared a light.
Light can be heard I know, because
When I first heard your voice,
Somehow instantly I knew
You were sent to help, God's choice.
The old me was a person
That you didn't choose to know.
You wrapped support around me

And helped me let him go.
With skill you planted just two seeds
Inside my ravaged mind.
Compassionately you nurtured them
With dedication of rare kind.
For endless hours, you worked with me
With caring I'd not seen,
Until again inside me grew
My hope and self-esteem.
Gently then you led the way
Over pebbles, stones, then rocks,
And firmly pushed me up the hills
With keys for all the locks.
Finally the wind of new
Refreshing on my face,
You pointed to the mountain tops
Where I should find my place.
As I stride toward that goal
I often pause in fear,
Cast, tentative, a backward glance,
Praying you're still near.
Looking o'er my shoulder
Again I see your wave,
Hear silently you telling me
You want me to be brave.
I know that I will make it,
Will build my life anew,
Attain at last that pinnacle,
Triumphant, thanks to you.
This new me has a purpose.
The care bestowed by you
I'll now dispense to others,
Then they can share it too!

A. Taylor, (1996), Reprinted with permission from: *The Journal of Cognitive Rehabilitation*, Vol. 14, Issue 5, p. 4.

REFERENCES

Bach-y-Rita, P. (1992). Recovery from brain damage. *Journal of Neuropsychological Rehabilitation, 6,* 191–199.

Bracy, O. (1994). *Soft-tools for cognitive rehabilitation,* Indianapolis: Neuroscience.

Bolger, J. F. (1980). Cognitive rehabilitation: A developmental approach. *Clinical Neuropsychology, 4,* 66–70.

Christensen, A-L. (1987). Rehabilitation planned in accordance with the Luria neuropsychological investigation: A case history of a patient with left sided aneurysm. *Neuropsychology, 1,* 45–48.

Cicerone, K. D. (1989). Psychotherapeutic interventions with traumatically brain-injured patients. *Rehabilitation Psychology, 34,* 105–114.

Gianutsos, R. (1991). Cognitive rehabilitation: A neuropsychological specialty comes of age. *Brain Injury, 5,* 353–368.

Klonoff, P. S., O'Brien, K. P., Prigatano, G. P., Chiapello, P. A., & Cunningham, M. (1989). Cognitive retraining after traumatic brain injury and its role in facilitating awareness. *Journal of Head Trauma Rehabilitation, 4,* 37–45.

Laatsch, L. (1983). Development of a memory training program. *Cognitive Rehabilitation, 1,* 15–19.

Laatsch, L. (1996). Benefits of integrating cognitive rehabilitation and psychotherapy in treatment of clients with neuropsychological impairments. *Journal of Cognitive Rehabilitation, 14,* 18–21.

Laatsch, L., Jobe, T., Synchra, J., Lin, Q., & Blend, M. (1997). Impact of CRT on neuropsychological impairments as measured by brain perfusion SPECT: A longitudinal study. *Brain Injury, 11,* 851–863.

Langer, K. G. (1992). Psychotherapy with the neuropsychologically-impaired adult. *American Journal of Psychotherapy, 46,* 620–639.

Langer, K. G., & Padrone, F. J. (1992). Psychotherapeutic treatment of awareness in acute rehabilitation of traumatic brain injury, *Neuropsychological Rehabilitation, 2,* 59–70.

Lehr, E. (1990). *Psychological management of traumatic brain injuries in children and adolescents.* Rockville, MD: Aspen.

Lewis, L. (1991). A framework for developing a psychotherapy treatment plan with brain-injured patients. *Journal of Head Trauma Rehabilitation, 6,* 22–29.

Lewis, L. (1992). Two neuropsychological models and their psychotherapeutic implications. *Bulletin of Menninger Clinic, 56,* 20–32.

Lewis, L., Athey, G., Eyman, J., & Saeks, S. (1992). Psychological treatment of adult psychiatric patients with traumatic frontal lobe injury. *Journal of Neuropsychiatry, 4,* 323–330.

Lewis, L., & Langer, K. G. (1994). Symbolization in psychotherapy with patients who are disabled. *American Journal of Psychotherapy, 48,* 231–239.

Lewis, L., & Rosenberg, S. J. (1990). Psychoanalytic psychotherapy with brained injured adult psychiatric patients. *Journal of Nervous and Mental Disease, 178,* 69–77.

Matthews, C., Harley, J., & Malec, J. (1987). Division 40: Task Force Report on Guidelines for Computer-assisted neuropsychological rehabilitation and cognitive remediation. *The Clinical Neuropsychologist, 2,* 161–184.

Mazmanian, P. E., Martin, K. O., & Kreutzer, J. S. (1991). Professional development and educational program planning in cognitive rehabilitation. In J. S. Kreutzer & P. H. Wehman (Eds.), *Cognitive rehabilitation for persons with traumatic brain injury: A functional approach* (pp. 35–51). Baltimore: P. H. Brooks.

Morris, J., & Bleiberg, J. (1986). Neuropsychological rehabilitation and traditional psychotherapy. *International Journal of Clinical Neuropsychology, 8,* 133–135.

National Head Injury Foundation (1989). *Interagency Head Injury Task Force Report,* Washington, DC: National Institute of Neurological Disorders and Stroke, NIH.

Parente, R., & Herrmann, D. (1996). *Retraining cognition: Techniques and applications.* Gaithersburg, MD: Aspen.

Prigatano, G. P. (1995). 1994 Sheldon Berrol, MD, Senior Lectureship: The problem of lost normality after brain injury. *Journal of Head Trauma Rehabilitation 10,* 87–95.

Prigatano, G. P., & Klonoff, P. S. (1988). Psychotherapy and neuropsychological assessment after brain injury. *Journal of Head Trauma Rehabilitation, 3,* 45–56.

Stern, J. M. (1985). The psychotherapeutic process with brain-injured patients: A dynamic approach. *Israel Journal of Psychiatry and Related Sciences, 22,* 83–87.

Taylor, R. (1996). From the patient's point of view. *Journal of Cognitive Rehabilitation, 14,* 4.

8.

Dealing with Rationalization and Unawareness in the Treatment of Visual Inattention

**Joseph Weinberg, Ph.D. and
Leonard Diller, Ph.D.**

INTRODUCTION

Unilateral spatial neglect is a disorder characterized by the patient's diminished response to stimuli on the side contralateral to the hemisphere lesion. It occurs more often in patients with right hemispheric damage than those with left hemispheric damage (Kinsbourne, 1993). A loss of visual field is often suffered but the person continues as if no loss has occurred.

The behavior of the patient with spatial neglect has been the subject of study and speculation over the past century. The disorder may be expressed in a variety of confusing ways from a failure to identify a limb as paralyzed to a lame excuse for difficulty in engaging in a normal activity such as reading a newspaper (Weinberg & Diller, 1968). Attempts have been made to identify the disturbance in association with locus of lesion (McGlinchey-Berroth et al., 1996); sensory diminishment (Battersby, Bender, Pollack, & Kahn, 1956; Gianutsos &

Mathesson, 1987); cerebral imbalance in processing information (Birch, Belmont, & Karp, 1967; Kinsbourne, 1993); a premorbid tendency to deny, minimize, or repress unpleasant events (Weinstein & Kahn, 1955); and a disturbance in dealing with informational complexity wherein individuals must infer information which is not experienced directly (Levine, 1990). Some have postulated a specific system of awareness which is impaired following brain injury (McGlynn & Schachter, 1989). Many tests have been developed over the past 50 years to capture and measure the patient's diminishment of space. The bulk of this literature aims to identify the nature and antecedents of this condition in order to increase our understanding. Such accounts may be useful in attempting to understand neglect, but leave open the question of how to approach the patient if one wishes to ameliorate the problem. Attempting to engage a person in a problem which is not acknowledged poses an active clinical issue for workers in a rehabilitation setting.

In this paper we pursue an important clinical issue in unawareness, common in cases of visual neglect, which must be considered from the perspective of the remediator. In order to engage the subject in problem solving or remediation, there must be a plausible reason for such engagement from the subject's perspective. The remediator's treatment scheme asks: How does the individual who is unaware interpret the situation? Is there a problem? If there is a problem what might be the reason for it? If the individual is unaware of a problem when it is pointed out, to what can he or she attribute deviant performance?

In psychiatric disorders and in everyday life, distorted attributions have been related to helplessness and depression and influence emotional and behavioral responses. In people without brain injury, distorted impressions due to misperceptions or faulty reasoning, excess drive may be driven by defense mechanisms. These serve as critical barriers to be removed in insight therapies ranging from psychoanalysis to cognitive behavioral therapies. The diminished awareness associated with neurologic disturbance calls forth defensive maneuvers which must be addressed before and during therapy. The defensive maneuvers which act to cover up feelings of shame when cognitive slippage appears, result in lack of engagement in rehabilitation therapies from perceptual retraining to ambulation retraining to participation in social groups. Clinically the most common presenting feature of a perceptual problem, therefore, is not the denial of a problem, but the defensive maneuver offered as a rationalization or excuse for failure. An example of such a maneuver would be the person who does not read a newspaper due to a perceptual problem who may say, "I can read, but I am not reading today because I forgot my glasses"; or "I am tired." In dealing with the problem the therapist must move rapidly to deal with the unawareness by rearranging situations and/or facts which will capture the patient's immediate attention. In a series of papers we outlined a number of strategies to facilitate remediation of the difficulty. The earlier papers include a set of training modules using principles and illustrations of anchoring, pacing, feedback, information load, and stimulus density (Weinberg et al., 1977, 1979; Weinberg, Piasetsky, Diller, & Gordon, 1982) to improve performance. More recently, we addressed the issue of resistant patients who pose problems in remediation. We argued that resistance, response style, and unawareness shared common features related to severity of cognitive impairment (Diller & Weinberg, 1993). Individuals who are unaware of a problem "resist" engagement in a therapeutic alliance. We suggested that unawareness is not a unitary all or nothing phenomenon, but exists in different degrees. The training situation could be greatly facilitated by taking into account the individual's response style. Response styles may be identified at four levels, ranging from active resistance to admit the presence of a stimulus, to indifferent passive denial when an error is pointed out, to passive denial accompanied by complexity when confronted by error, to ready acknowledgment of a problem without the necessary action to correct it. Knowledge of response style is a key to an individual's level of unawareness and provides the remediator with clues regarding stimuli and strategies for treatment, as well as guides for duration and outcome. Briefly, the more unaware the individual, the more simple the program, the more modest the goals, and the longer the expected duration of treatment will be.

Our experiences are based on therapeutic contacts, generally on a weekly basis, with over 100 patients over the past 20 years. We noted patient accounts of their problems and their treatment. In this paper we present case studies which may serve as useful paradigms for clinical interventions. We selected two patients with markedly restricted awareness of their failures or at least limited willingness to admit failure, to illustrate how resistant patients can be engaged in treatment. These patients had completed a course of physical and occupational therapy and had reached a plateau in these areas. Their perceptual–cognitive problems alarmed their families and caused them to seek further help.

CASE 1

Mr. A, a successful 68-year-old professional, sustained a right parietal embolic infarct. Initial psychological evaluation revealed perceptual problems manifested by a left neglect and impulsiveness, a left-sided facial weakness, and a left-sided numbness. As an inpatient in a rehabilitation program it was noted that Mr. A was aware of what had happened to him, but unaware of residual cognitive impairments. The report read: "He remains unaware of cognitive changes and the implications of his condition. He plans to return to work, with no insight into the potential changes caused by his disability." A summary of the neuropsychological examination at 4 months postonset, when he was transferred to an outpatient program, found problems in attention and concentration and in visuomotor functioning. While verbal scores were above average, perceptual performance was significantly impaired (Verbal IQ = 117; Performance IQ = 74). Attention to details in the visual environment, sequential visuomotor activities, activities requiring organization of information into meaningful or abstract wholes, and visual scanning accuracy, were markedly reduced, particularly as materials become more difficult.

When first seen for perceptual cognitive retraining, Mr. A avoided looking to his left when asked a question by the interviewer. He asserted that his only problems were residual physical difficulties and memory failure in recalling names. He had been told that he had a short-term memory problem based on his performance on the neuropsychological examination. He also complained of "being tired." When pressed about his cognitive problem, he remarked that he first had such problems immediately after his stroke, but they cleared after a couple of weeks "just as my speech came back and my right side came back." He felt that his attention and concentration were no different than before the stroke. The main problems were memory and fatigue (see Table 8.1).

In the first working session he was instructed to ask the therapist as to the purpose of any task which was to be given to him. He was told that periodically he would be questioned about his problems and the rationale for any exercises that were assigned. He was told that he should know about and be able to explain the exercises. Because he was not fully aware of the nature of his perceptual problems, by verbalizing the reasons for the exercises, his awareness and understanding of his problems would be enhanced and this would help him engage in ways to deal with them.

He received a task involving simple multiplications (see Figure 8.1). As the figure illustrates, he failed to deal with the number "5" in the first problem and the number "9" in the second problem. He was told that the difficulty was not in multiplication, since he multiplied numbers correctly, but rather in the neglect of the left side of space. He was surprised that he omitted the numbers 5 in the first problem and 9 in the second problem. "How much space do the numbers take up?" he remarked. He also received a visual cancellation task and the Weinberg "and, the, but" task (Diller and Weinberg, 1993). Difficulties in scanning to the left and attention and concentration were pointed out (for a description of the problem and the remedial strategies see Table 8.1).

In one hour a week training sessions and 15 minutes a day of home exercises, he improved in visual scanning. As treatment progressed, exercises were increased to 30 to 45 minutes

TABLE 8.1
Description of Problems and Remedial Techniques

Description of Problems	Remedial Techniques
A. Patient Unaware that He Has a Problem	Given arithmetical calculation such as 543 × 345. Task can't be rationalized
B. Patient Does Not Look to the Left, Head Tilted to the Right	1. Explain to patient the importance of looking at faces while communicating with others (e.g., "Look at me") 2. Practice moving head to the center, then to the left
C. Patient Has Difficulty Scanning to the Left of Side of Sphere	1. Following finger moving from left to right.[a] 2. Looking at index cards attached on a wall (left to right side). 3. Crossing out letter/letters. 4. Copying first and last word.
D. Increasing Patient's Attention	1. Canceling words: *and, the, but,* in editorials. 2. Serial numerical task to increase attention over time and increase attentional load.[b]
E. Reading	1. Summarizing short articles (written). 2. Reading popular magazine articles and summarizing: oral and written.
F. Arithmetic	Practice arithmetical subtraction & multiplications 2 × 2, 3 × 2, 4 × 2, etc.

[a] Instructions: "Move finger L to R, if patient fails, repeat. If fails again, discontinue. If pass, use index fingers of both hands moving parallel.

[b] Written serial numerical task—modifying information load; e.g., add serial 3's—3, 6, 9; serial 5's—5, 10, 15; 3 & 5's, $3 + 5 = 8$, $+ 3 = 11$, $+ 15 = 26$, etc. A similar principle is used for serial subtraction. From $700 -$ subtract 3's, then subtract 7's, then combine alternating 3's and 7's.

Figure 8.1. Arithmetic performance: Mr. A & Mr. Z.

Mr. A

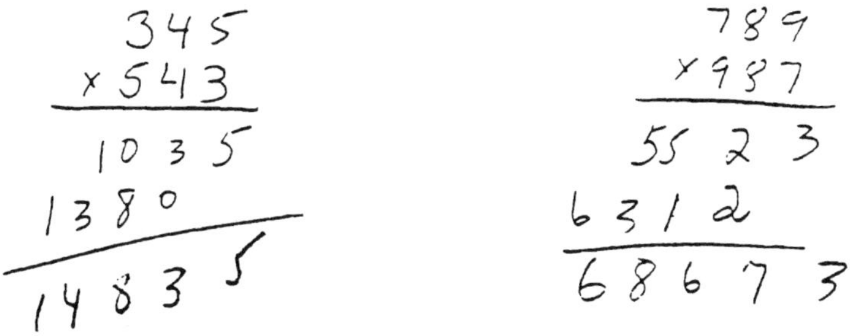

$$
\begin{array}{r}
345 \\
\times 543 \\
\hline
1035 \\
1380 \\
\hline
14835
\end{array}
\qquad
\begin{array}{r}
789 \\
\times 987 \\
\hline
5523 \\
6312 \\
\hline
68673
\end{array}
$$

Mr. Z

$$
\begin{array}{r}
456 \\
\times 534 \\
\hline
1824 \\
1368 \\
\hline
1504
\end{array}
\qquad
\begin{array}{r}
789 \\
\times 897 \\
\hline
5523 \\
716 \\
6312 \ 33 \\
\hline
107763
\end{array}
$$

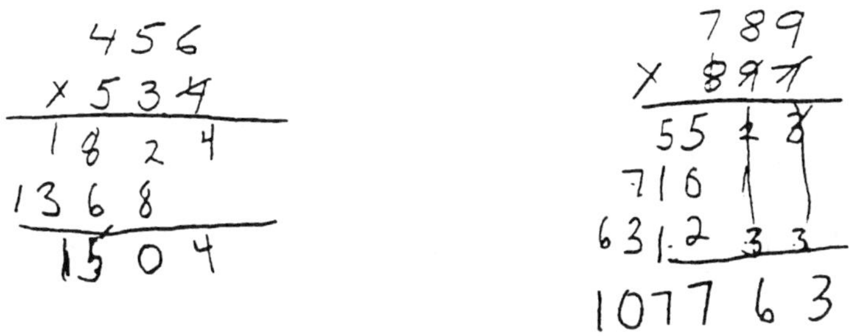

per day. After 12 sessions, Mr. A returned to his office on a part-time basis, and after 24 sessions he returned on a full-time basis. He continued the exercises for 3 months. He is now actively involved in his work, travels, and participates in his social life. Below is an account of how Mr A summarized his training.

First I could not understand why I could not resume my work and drive a car. Although I was told that I sustained a neglect of visual space and had cognitive problems, I could not relate these problems to daily activities. I was also told that I was improving and yet I was told that I had cognitive problems. I was confused and so was my family. . . . In the training sessions, my problems and the ways they were affecting my thinking and organization, were pointed out to me. When I left out numbers in multiplication or when asked to cancel the words *and, the, but* in an editorial column and saw the number of my omissions, the neglect problem became clearer to me. I could not dismiss or fail to see the impact on my daily activities. My attention and concentration improved, and I was able to stay with a task for longer periods of time without getting tired. I was able to accept an explanation for my difficulties in reading newspapers and watching television. Avoiding movies, which I excused as "I am tired," was related to attention and concentration and not lack of interest.

I was told (and this was reinforced by my family) that I was depressed and not motivated. This was difficult for me to accept. Before the stroke I was active in projects and was too busy to be depressed. During rehabilitation, I was deprived of normal activities which reenforced the impression that I was depressed.

CASE 2

Mr. Z is a 52-year-old, right-handed social scientist who sustained a right CVA. On neurological evaluation he manifested a left hemianopsia and a left hemipegia. A CT scan revealed an edema and a mass involving the right temporal and parietal lobes.

Five months postonset he was admitted to the outpatient department of the Rusk Institute of Rehabilitation Medicine. Neuropsychological evaluation showed a significant loss of intelligence from a pretraumatic level. Deficits in visual processing, visual memory, planning, and cognitive flexibility appeared, as well as problems in attention, concentration, reading, arithmetic skills (Verbal IQ = 138; Performance IQ = 65). When presented with a newspaper, he read headlines only on the right side of the page. He skipped lines and had difficulty in making sense of what he read. Similarly, in copying, he copied only the right side of the page, omitting the left. Attention to visual details was profoundly impaired.

When first seen for cognitive retraining, Mr. Z was asked a sequence of questions: whether he had a problem in visual perception, whether he was omitting objects on the left, how he was perceiving his problem, why he was referred for therapy. His main concerns were with physical motor skills such as walking, lack of independence, and inability to drive (Table 8.2).

TABLE 8.2
Perceived Problems of Patients

	Mr. A	Mr. Z
What is your problem?	1. Difficulty Walking	Can't Walk
	2. Lacks Independence	Lacks Independence
	3. Can't Drive	Can't Drive
	4. Can't Travel	Can't Travel
Did you read paper before?	Yes	Yes
Do you read paper now?	No. Why? Hard to hold. Not interested in news	Not like before stroke; I have no patience
Do you have a reading problem?	No	No
Reading or understanding what is read?	No	No
Do you watch TV?	Yes	Yes
Understand TV?	No problem	No problem
Do you have problems with vision or seeing things?	No No	M.D. says I have problems (hasn't seen eye doctor in 2 years)
Do you have a problem with attention or concentration?	Memory . . . can't remember	Short-term memory . . . "tend to forget now & then, so I'm told"

During the brief interview, he did not look at the examiner, who was seated to his left. He looked to the right or at the floor. On command he looked at the interviewer. During a 50-minute session, 22 times he was told to look to the left. According to the patient, he had no problem in reading professional journals, despite the fact that he omitted half of the newspaper headlines. The reason he was referred to cognitive retraining was to improve his ambulation and driving.

Before engaging in retraining it was necessary to confront Mr. Z with the presence of his visual perceptual problem and his neglect, and how these problems pervaded his academic activities and interfered with his judgments and social contacts. As in the case of Mr. A, previously cited, arithmetic calculation served as a primary therapeutic vehicle, with similar results (Figure 8.1). When omission of digits in performing calculations was pointed out, Mr. Z stated that he had not performed simple calculations in a long time and, indeed, in the following session he brought a calculator to prove his point. When it was noted that the purpose of the exercise was not to illustrate an arithmetic difficulty but a visual perceptual problem, he suggested that he could set up a formula to make it easier to multiply 3×3 and 3×4. While it was possible that he neglected stimuli on the left side of space, he argued that this did not affect his profession and his general behavior. Although he improved and learned to compensate for his neglect, as did Mr. A, he continued to rationalize all failures, offering reasons for his difficulties. For example, he brought a paper that he was reviewing for a scientific journal. When asked to read the summary, he left out words on the left side and skipped lines. When these errors were pointed out, he commented that the omitted words and the skipped lines were unimportant. He remarked that when he had difficulty with a task and saw the reason why he failed, he committed himself and needed to have a reason for the failure even if it did not make sense to others.

Mr. Z improved and learned to compensate for the neglect and difficulties in scanning. On the Weinberg "and, the, but" test he omitted 41 of 48 targets initially. On retest, after 2 months of training, he omitted only three targets, placing him within the normal range. He continued training for 3 months, feeling comfortable with his progress, before he discontinued treatment.

DISCUSSION

In our earlier studies we developed methods, principles, and evidence for an approach to perceptual remediation for visual neglect. These efforts parallel developments in psychotherapy research which culminated in manuals used in clinical trials to demonstrate efficacy of treatment (Garfield, 1997). Such an approach is congruent with requests of third-party payers for evidence before treatment is reimbursed. However, psychotherapy researchers who note limitations in this approach, when describing experiences in applying the manuals in clinical trials, ascribe such limitations to individual differences in the use of these manuals by training therapists (Beutler, 1997). That is, for a given clinician a manual may be quite effective for one patient but not for another (Strupp & Anderson, 1997). In a sense, in this paper we have taken a step back from previous writings. We have shown the interplay between what is generally considered as clinical sensitivity to patient response through examples of situations that are generally not reported in formal studies. We report the clinical fine tuning that goes along with formal procedures.

In presenting materials to deal with unawareness in Table 8.1, we note that depending on the clinical situation, it is often useful to start with naturalistic situations or common stimuli which are part of conventional surroundings. For example, ask a patient to describe a picture on a wall and note omissions in the description. Note whether or not the patient looks at the examiner during an interview or conversation, or point out discrepancies in grooming or appearance. This is also useful in the presence of a significant other. The examiner calls the patient's attention to these problems with gentle probes: "Why do you think you omitted this or why do you think I gave you this task in the first place or how do you think you appear to others?" The remediator's feedback is very specific to the patient's response to the given task to ensure that the reason for the failure is not falsely generalized ("I'm dumb!") or falsely attributed ("I have a memory problem or I am not wearing my glasses!"). The remediator might say, "You may have failed to notice the details in the picture not because you are dumb or careless or mentally incompetent or nearsighted, but because since your stroke you find it easier to pay attention to one space over the other. You are simply following your old prestroke habits. Let me show you a way around the problem."

The remediator illustrates or models ways in which perceptual habits can be altered to overcome the problems, and offers ways in which retraining can be helpful. Casting the response so specifically, followed by corrective action which is equally specific, gives the patient the feeling of working with someone who understands and accepts his problem and can deal with it in an open way without the patient feeling diminished. One of the obstacles in treatment is the patient's feelings of shame as a result of failure or fear of failure on seemingly simple tasks.

The strategy helps restore a patient's sense of mastery and reduces feelings of shame. It is common for patients to give priority to this treatment over other forms of therapies, even though in rehabilitation it is more typical for patients to prefer building functional motor skills. Thus patients may request this treatment after being discharged from the remainder of rehabilitation therapies.

In a previous paper (Diller & Weinberg, 1993) we noted that patients with low levels of awareness resist acknowledging problems even on direct confrontation and in the face of overwhelming evidence. We argued that acknowledgment and engagement can be facilitated by presenting the patient with samples of behavior which were difficult to deny (e.g., having to read one's own handwriting, or reviewing omissions in an important overlearned task such as making change with coins which are spread on the table). In the cases of Mr. A and Mr. Z, we illustrate the same effect by the use of simple arithmetic as a sample of behavior to enhance awareness of difficulties, in that arithmetic is a necessary overlearned skill which is meaningful. Unlike reading, where the person can fill in the meaning of omitted words, the consequences of failure are readily apparent. An important step is to show the patient strategies for overcoming the failures on the spot. The key element is that the failure does not have to result in a loss of personal control. Much of the attempt to cover up or deny a problem is to hide embarrassment over failure in ordinary events. Often the embarrassment is not presented on initial contact and appears only with more close contact and trust. Mr. A's case illustrates the feeling of regaining mastery. Mr. Z's case illustrates the struggle to retain mastery. He attempts to retain mastery over each situation anew.

In this paper, we also illustrate the rationalizations of both patients, steps taken to correct the rationalizations by systematic verbalization of the presence of the problem, explanation of steps taken to overcome it, and concrete success in finding the correct solution. The rationalizations are illustrated in Table 8.2 and the sequence of tasks used to bring out the problem and correct it in Table 8.1. The rationalizations present only a sample of situations. For example, a patient may avoid social engagements because of embarrassment in not recognizing people, while insisting that he doesn't go out because he is not interested. In rationalizations it is important that one deal directly, yet tactfully with the stated reason and correct it. For example, when Mr. A said that he had a memory problem but not a perceptual problem, he was asked what he had eaten the night before. Upon answering correctly, he was told that there was evidence of good working memory, but the problem was perceptual. Memory difficulties, a common reason offered for failure, serve as an excuse for not addressing a treatable problem.

Although the unawareness had its roots in visual dysfunction, unawareness occurs in a variety of situations with brain injured individuals, which are not due to stroke and are not associated with visual difficulties. Rationalizations for failure may involve similar defensive maneuvers and would call into play similar therapeutic strategies. The syndromes described here are more striking and the strategies can be explicated more clearly.

It is also apparent that awareness and success in perceptual retraining does not occur suddenly or by leaps and bounds. Because perceptual problems are pervasive and recur in unexpected as well as expected situations, rationalizations are frequently invoked until the person learns to identify the reasons for failure.

One note. Mr. A stated how unhappy he was because of his initial confusion. Both family and staff attributed this to depression as a more pervasive condition. While Mr. A may have been depressed, it is useful to distinguish and treat the elements which enter into depression rather than considering it as a blanket affective state. While some have attributed depression to biological factors (Robinson et al., 1981), we have noted that limitations of normal activity patterns are highly correlated with depression (Gordon et al., 1985). The reasons for the depression and different patterns of treatment are beyond the scope of this chapter.

REFERENCES

Battersby, W. J., Bender, M. B., Pollack, M., & Kahn, R. L. (1956). Unilateral "spatial agnosia" (inattention) in patients with cerebral lesions. *Brain, 79,* 68–92.

Beutler, L. (1997). The psychotherapist as a neglected variable in psychotherapy: An illustration by reference to the role of the therapist experience and training. *Clinical Psychology, 4,* 44–53.

Birch, H. G., Belmont, I., & Karp, E. (1967). Delayed information processing and extinction following cerebral damage. *Brain, 90,* 113–130.

Diller, L., & Weinberg, J. (1993). Response styles in perceptual retraining. In W. A. Gordon (Ed.), *Advances in stroke rehabilitation* (pp. 162–182). Andover, MD: Andover Press.

Garfield, S. L. (1997). The therapist as a neglected variable in psychotherapy research. *Clinical Psychology, 4,* 40–43.

Gianutsos, R., & Mathesson, P. (1987). The rehabilitation of visual perceptual disorders attributable to brain injury. In M. J. Meier, A. Benton, & L. Diller (Eds.), *Neuropsychological rehabilitation* (pp. 202–241). New York: Churchill-Livingston.

Gordon, W. A., Hibbard, M. R., Egelko, S., Shaver, M. S., Leiberman, A., & Ragnarsson, K. (1985). Perceptual remediation in patients with right brain damage: A comprehensive program. *Archives of Physical Medicine and Rehabilitation, 66,* 353–359.

Kinsbourne, M. (1993). Orientational bias model of unilateral neglect: Evidence from attentional gradients within hemispace. In I. H. Robertson & J. C. Marshall (Eds.), *Unilateral neglect: Clinical and experimental studies* (pp. 63–86). Hove, U.K.: Lawrence Erlbaum.

Levine, D. (1990). Unawareness of visual and sensorimotor defects: A hypothesis. *Brain and Cognition, 13,* 233–281.

McGlynn, S. M., & Schachter, D. L. (1989). Unawareness of deficits in neuropsychological syndromes. *Journal of Clinical and Experimental Neuropsychology, 11,* 143–205.

McGlynchey-Berroth, R., Bullis, D. P., Milberg, W. P., Verfaellie, M., Alexander, M., & D'Esposito, M. (1996). Assessment of neglect reveals dissociable behavioral but not anatomical subtypes. *Journal of the International Neuropsychology Society, 2,* 441–451.

Robinson, R. G., Kubos, K. L., Starr, L. K., Rao, K., & Price, T. (1981). Mood changes in stroke patients: Relationship to locus of lesion. *American Journal of Psychiatry, 24,* 555–566.

Strupp, H. H., & Anderson, T. (1997). On limitations of therapy manuals. *Clinical Psychology, 4,* 76–82.

Weinberg, J., & Diller, L. (1968). *On reading newspapers by hemiplegics: Denial of a visual disability.* Paper presented at the 76th Annual Meeting of the American Psychological Association, San Francisco, CA.

Weinberg, J., Diller, L., Gordon, W. A, Gerstman, L. J., Leiberman, A., Lakin, P., Hodges, G., & Ezrachi, O. (1977). Visual scanning training effect on reading-related tasks in acquired right brain damage. *Archives of Physical Medicine and Rehabilitation 59,* 491–496.

Weinberg, J., Diller, L., Gordon, W. A., Gerstman, L. J., Leiberman, A., Lakin, P., Hodges, G., & Ezrachi, O. (1979). Training sensory awareness and spatial organization in people with right brain damage. *Archives of Physical Medicine and Rehabilitation, 60,* 491–496.

Weinberg, J., Piasetsky, E., Diller, L., & Gordon, W. A. (1982). Treating perceptual organization deficits in nonneglecting RBD stroke patients. *Journal of Clinical Neuropsychology, 4,* 59–75.

Weinstein, E. A., & Kahn, R. L. (1955). *The denial of illness.* Springfield, IL: Charles C Thomas.

PART IV

Specialized Treatment Applications for Specific Population Needs

9.

Group Psychotherapy

Donna M. Langenbahn, Ph.D.,
Rose Lynn Sherr, Ph.D.,
Dvorah Simon, Ph.D.,
and Bennett Hanig, Ph.D.

OVERVIEW

This chapter is based upon our experiences working with adults with brain injury in a large outpatient neuropsychology program. The Neuropsychology Service (NPS) of the Psychology Department of the Rusk Institute of Rehabilitation Medicine annually provides cognitive and psychotherapeutic services to approximately 250 adult outpatients with acquired neuropsychological impairment (Sherr & Langenbahn, 1992). Both cognitive and psychosocial group treatment are integral to the NPS treatment approach. Our clinical experiences and those of others have indicated the value of group treatment with this population, used both alone and integrated with individual treatment (e.g., Ben-Yishay & Diller, 1981; Deaton, 1991; Prigatano et al., 1986).

Group treatment can both intensify and extend the benefits obtained from individual treatment for brain injured individuals. Groups provide the opportunity for peer support and feedback, the sharing of effective ideas and compensatory strategies, the sense of feeling helpful, the easing of isolation, and repeated comparisons of one's abilities and limitations with those of others with the same or a similar diagnosis.

The potential benefits of group treatment address one of the general goals of psychotherapy with individuals with brain injury, i.e., to assist with the emotional and social changes that make their lives so difficult following the injury. However, the brain injury also results in cognitive, emotional, and social changes that may render traditional approaches to psychotherapy ineffective. Skills such as attention and concentration, verbal expression and comprehension, memory, cognitive flexibility, generalization, empathy, and abstract thinking are thought to be essential for effective psychological treatment; yet these capabilities can be impaired by brain injury (e.g., Miller, 1993, pp. 54–67). Further, brain injury can cause reduced ability to be aware of, observe, and monitor one's feelings, thoughts, and actions (Prigatano & Schacter, 1991), also essential capacities for effective psychotherapy. The resulting array of limitations often engenders a new and confusing sense of "self." Concurrently, one's capacity to stabilize oneself with what Weiner (1966) referred to as consistent and organized patterns of dealing with people, affects, and life situations is often drastically reduced.

MODIFICATIONS IN PSYCHOTHERAPY AFTER BRAIN INJURY

In general, psychotherapy is adapted to meet the needs and abilities of the individual(s) being treated. To treat the brain injured individual in a group setting, two other critical adaptations of traditional psychotherapy need to be considered: (1) the ways in which psychotherapy must be altered to provide comfort and to make change possible for the brain injured individual; (2) the methods that allow individuals with brain injury to participate meaningfully in group psychotherapeutic treatment. Successful realization of both adaptations involve a knowledge of brain injury based difficulties as they impact on the individual's ability to benefit from psychotherapeutic interventions.

With regard to the first consideration, rehabilitation literature now reflects the commonly accepted viewpoint that individual psychotherapy must be modified for brain injured individuals (Langer, 1992; Lewis & Rosenberg, 1990; Prigatano et al., 1986). Miller (1993) enlarges the scope of modifications considerably:

> Psychotherapy, in the broadest sense, may include remedial instruction, specialized training, manipulation and structuring of the environment, medication where appropriate, and supportive, behavioral, cognitive, and psychodynamic approaches to psychotherapy. (p. 48)

Our experience suggests that many approaches and techniques used in cognitive remediation also must be incorporated into the practice of psychotherapy, both individual and group, in order for persons with brain injury to benefit optimally (Ben-Yishay & Diller, 1981; Sherr & Langenbahn, 1992).

Specific modifications include a set of procedures and techniques that transform the psychotherapy in line with an overall approach with this population: repetition; checking the patient's comprehension of what has been said; the consideration of cognitive hypotheses for behaviors commonly interpreted as dynamically based "resistance" (e.g., poor eye contact, lateness, moments of forgetting). Written notes are used either by, or, if necessary, for the patient within sessions along with reviewing within sessions and journal-keeping outside of sessions. The therapist utilizes diagrams, drawings, checklists, graphs, and other methods of concretizing information and ideas. The pace of treatment is slowed. Scaling or rating techniques are used for anchoring experience of difficulties, viewing difficulties on a continuum, and measuring change. Normalizing frames of reference are used for both injury and noninjury related experience. Therapeutic interventions are altered based upon the understanding that cognitive/perceptual difficulties can trigger defensive reactions (e.g., difficulties in auditory comprehension may evoke symptoms of regression, obsessiveness, or denial), and, conversely, defensive reactions can exacerbate cognitive or perceptual difficulties (e.g., obsessiveness can reduce attentional focus).

In order for individuals with brain injury to benefit from group treatment, the approach mentioned above must be adapted further. Yalom (1985) notes that group psychotherapy is a guided encounter in which the therapist sets up the environment and format of the group to promote certain "therapeutic factors" (e.g., cohesiveness, universality, and interpersonal relationship). These therapeutic factors are not easily attainable with a brain injured population due to cognitive compromise and the impairment of more basic social and emotional abilities. Thus, the initial focus of group psychotherapy with this population often must entail the rebuilding of basic underlying social skills as much as possible, and then, practice in the management of emotional reactions within the context of varying reductions in ego defensive and cognitive capacities. Structuring techniques of group interaction (i.e., instructions, cues, modeling, and other explicit information) may also be used to guide group members so they can participate successfully in group interaction and generalize the benefits gained to their everyday lives.

PSYCHOSOCIAL IMPACT OF NEUROPSYCHOLOGICAL IMPAIRMENT

Neuropsychological impairment after brain injury reduces psychosocial functioning in very basic ways. For instance, significant deficits in cognitive areas such as the ability to think abstractly may create problems in taking another's perspective, in seeing oneself accurately in interpersonal situations, and in understanding social context, boundaries, timing, and distance. Often observed, also, is a certain "narcissism," not necessarily based on psychodynamic etiology, but related to the above-mentioned difficulties.

For those with severe cognitive impairments, a loss of friends and social contacts might be noted, but the causes are often attributed to others' lack of understanding. Feelings of anger (often compounded due to emotional disinhibition), anxiety, and depression, as well as further social withdrawal, often worsen rather than rectify the situation. Severe impairments in initiation can reduce access to constructive preinjury behaviors, including those necessary in developing and maintaining social relationships and activities.

Individuals with only moderate impairment of such cognitive abilities as abstract reasoning show social–emotional functioning characterized by relatively greater flexibility of thought and reason. Greater perspective, capacity for self-assessment, and ability to acknowledge personal contributions to emotional and social well-being may still be present. Most importantly, there is more ability to acknowledge the need to change one's own behavior to improve social and emotional dysfunction. With those having moderate cognitive impairment, while there may be an awareness of and discomfort with social isolation and dysfunction, the degree of cognitive limitation often still interferes with spontaneous remediative behaviors that are predicated upon social facility, initiation, and planning and organizational abilities.

Individuals with relatively minor changes in cognitive ability (presuming good premorbid social, emotional, and intellectual resources) usually have greater residual emotional and social capacity. They can acknowledge and label emotional experience, shift their perspective, hear feedback about the impact of their behavior upon others, and express empathy for and concern about others' experiences. While social functioning is commonly reduced from preinjury levels, the capacity to plan and implement social and recreational activities usually is retained. With increased cognitive capacity, there is greater general concern about emotional and interpersonal changes. Personal responsibility in the maintenance of friends and friendships is acknowledged. If the person is married or in a sustained intimate relationship, the preservation of that relationship, as well as the understanding of and adjustment to new roles and the resolution of conflict within the relationship, are central concerns.

GROUP TREATMENT OF PSYCHOLOGICAL AND PSYCHOSOCIAL PROBLEMS

General Rationale for Group Structure

The Neuropsychology Service has developed different types of groups addressing several aspects of psychological and psychosocial functioning. They include Psychosocial Groups, focusing on issues of social interaction and presentation of self; Self-Regulation Groups, dealing with emotional disruption of the process of logical thinking; and Anger Management Groups, for those whose loss of anger control has been identified as a significant problem by themselves, family members, friends, or staff.

Different protocols of treatment have been developed within each type of group to accommodate differences in the level of preinjury life experience, developmental level and intelligence, and extent of cognitive impairment. Modifications are designed also to circumvent the effects of the brain injury so that maximum benefit can be derived from the treatment. Structuring techniques in psychotherapy groups include explicit determination and ongoing review of short- and long-term goals, the use of notetaking, following a prepared agenda, and reviewing of the previous session. Such techniques provide organization, memory compensation, and focus to the groups' activities. Based on the degree of impairment of group members, topics are made more or less limited or concrete, pace of group activities and discussions is slowed or quickened, repetition of key points is frequent or rare, and generalization exercises are emphasized or not. In addition to the group culture-building techniques described by Yalom (1985), responsibility for the group process is encouraged by group members taking charge of timekeeping, leading selected sections or exercises within groups, reviewing the previous session, and summarizing individual progress toward goals within sessions.

In the following sections, we will discuss the format and content of Psychosocial, Self-Regulation, and Anger Management Groups. Within each section, we will describe member selection issues, group format, and the details of treatment interventions.

Psychosocial Groups

Within the NPS program, Psychosocial Groups (PSs) are a subset of the Basic Skill Groups (BSGs) that comprise a large component of outpatient treatment (Sherr & Langenbahn, 1992). Training within BSGs emphasizes competence in five basic skills: awareness of current strengths and limitations; ability to pay attention to and concentrate on a task; effective use of notetaking for organizing and remembering information; the ability to give, accept, and use feedback as a means of self-evaluation; and emotional–social interaction skills. Individuals are assigned to BSGs by virtue of their level of competence in the five skill areas, as well as their overall residual intellect, speed of language and information processing, motivation, stamina, and tolerance for group interaction. Consideration is also given to factors of group cohesion (Yalom, 1985), such as age, education, and cultural background. However, group members are not necessarily separated by etiology of the brain injury. By use of neuropsychological data, clinical interview, and input from the brain injured individual, family, and treating staff, these factors are combined to result in "low," "moderate," and "high" level BSGs. These divisions are clinically useful to patients, who often have limited tolerance for seeing themselves as similar to more impaired individuals, or alternatively, experience anxiety in the face of group exercises that are too challenging, or other group members who have notably stronger cognitive abilities.

Psychosocial Groups, although a subset of BSGs in the NPS program, may be developed in any brain injury program in which the treatment of emotional and social interaction difficulties is essential. Despite the emotional and social interactive emphasis, PGs are introduced to members as distinct from traditional "psychotherapy" groups, in part to prevent the groups from being seen as open forums for complaints and "expressing feelings." Because individuals with brain injury often lack

control over emotional expression and have difficulty recognizing suitable contexts and the social consequences of unbridled
expression of thoughts and emotion, interactions in PGs first
highlight the educative and rational components in emotional
management and social exchange.

The initial focus in PGs is on the establishment of individualized goals, and groups emphasize achievement of these goals
throughout subsequent sessions. Although complaints and expression of feelings occur, group leaders seek to guide and
channel these, and other group phenomena, into reasoned
and effective communication and behavior. Psychosocial
Groups emphasize three of the five BSG skills noted above:
awareness of current strengths and limitations (especially in
emotional and social areas); ability to give, accept, and use
feedback as a means of self-evaluation; and improvement of
social interaction skills and management of emotional reactions.

Levels of Psychosocial Groups

We have found it useful to divide Psychosocial Groups into
three levels, depending upon individuals' cognitive and social
skill capabilities. The first, level 1, is designed to accommodate
the most psychosocially and cognitively impaired individuals.
Level 1 employs a highly structured approach (borrowed from
BSG cognitive remediation groups) in which sheets listing
group members' individual psychosocial goals are used, notetaking is stressed, and repetition is the norm. Level 1 PGs are
designed to focus on the basic building blocks of social skills
and awareness of social skill strengths and difficulties. These
building blocks include initiation of interpersonal interaction,
listening to others, modulation of voice volume and rate of
speech, speaking with animation and inflection, making appropriate eye contact, understanding body language, and planning
recreational (although not necessarily "social") outings.

Level 1 members also work on developing awareness of
their social skill limitations, giving and accepting feedback in
social skill areas, and developing means of judging their own

behavior in social situations. Interaction between and among group members is guided by highly structured exercises and is accompanied by monitoring and coaching from the group leader. Role playing and structured presentations frequently are used in level 1 groups, with goals and feedback centering around the skills mentioned above.

Level 2 groups are characterized by a moderate to high degree of structure that allows for a greater degree of interpersonal interaction among group members. While participants continue to work on the basic social skills mentioned above, more emphasis is placed on the development of social rapport, as well as on the sharpening of social judgment and problem solving. More emotionally-based goals are included in goal-setting in level 2 groups (e.g., self-acceptance, heightening of self-confidence, and reduction of social anxiety). After exhibiting competence in level 1 skills, patients in level 2 focus on the awareness of context and timing that heightens success in social interactions. Role-playing and structured presentations are also used in level 2 groups, with the goal of learning and practicing effective behavior in a variety of social situations.

Level 3 groups are for those functioning at the highest level of premorbid and current abilities. These individuals are generally reasonably aware of some of the implications of their cognitive deficits. They can interact socially with a moderate level of effectiveness, and they have the capacity to explore, acknowledge, and use feedback about their emotional reactions and social interactions.

Level 3 PGs are conducted with a low to moderate degree of structure. Typical goals include improving interpersonal skills, facilitating closer relationships within the group, heightening self-confidence, reducing social impulsivity, stabilizing mood, reducing social anxiety, developing greater insight into personality and interaction style, compensating for ineffective social behaviors, and working toward self-acceptance. Group goals can be achieved with less structured interaction among members, as well as more member input, as feedback from level 3 group participants often has a meaning and accuracy surpassing that in lower level groups. In level 3 PGs, the leader often acts more as a facilitator, but during certain exercises, still may give explicit and detailed instructions and feedback to assist in effective and emotionally safe group interactions. Treatment tools include role-play and semistructured discussions and presentations within topic areas selected by the leaders or by the group members.

Format of Psychosocial Groups

All Psychosocial Groups have the following format: (1) announcements; (2) review of previous session; (3) psychosocial exercise/discussion; and (4) summary of today's learning/progress. All groups use individualized goal sheets to record each member's personal goals. Videotaping is used to demonstrate successes and persistent problems, and to monitor improvement.

In all levels of PGs, isolation and repeated practice of the basic components of a task are accomplished before attempting the entire task. Suitable amounts of instruction, cuing, and feedback are provided depending upon the competence level of the group. This structured approach allows limited degrees of freedom for "errors," and thus promotes greater opportunity for success in performing exercises (Ben-Yishay, Diller, Gerstman, & Garden, 1970). With increased competence of group members, structure and cuing can be gradually reduced. Increased structure is often reintroduced for new goal areas, or when the task is made more complex by adding greater cognitive or interpersonal demands.

Announcements are brief; they include an account of who is present or absent, a reminder to refer to personal goals, mention of any planned absences for the following week, and examples of any successes or problems encountered in goal areas during the past week. In level 1 and 2 groups, group members often need structured guidelines in order to provide an example of a psychosocial success or a problem. Guidelines may be such as the following:

> An example gives enough information to paint a "mind picture," in an example you mention: (1) the goal for which you're giving the example; (2) where you were; (3) who was there; (4)

what happened; and (5) what body language and words you used to meet your goal.

Reviews in PGs focus on updating group members on the topics and principles learned in the previous session. Members are expected to have notes that assist them in presenting an informative overview of the previous session, and feedback is given primarily upon style of presentation, while also noting any major errors or omissions. The group leader adds comments, as needed.

In the psychosocial exercise/discussion section, the topic or exercise of the day is introduced. In level 1 and 2 groups, the exercise is highly or moderately structured, with clear instructions. In level 3 groups, the section may either be an exercise with moderate to low structure, or a guided discussion of a topic area. In the latter groups, while instructions may give more latitude for spontaneous responses, they are still designed to provide clarity about the group task.

In the final section of PGs, a brief summary of the session is given by a group member or group leader. Each member then evaluates the degree of personal learning and objective progress made toward individual goals in that day's session. Methods of assessing progress include use of rating scales to anchor observations from self, other group members, and group leader(s), listing of "principles" that can be practiced in everyday settings, and assistance in setting the next more challenging goal as progress is shown.

Exercises and Approaches

Initial sessions of all levels of Psychosocial Groups include discussions of the group and its purpose. The format for the orientation discussion varies according to the level of the group, but always involves concrete examples of the psychosocial problems that the therapy will address. In the higher level PGs, members are encouraged to bring in examples from their recent experience.

Levels 1 and 2. As noted earlier, goals addressed in level 1 PGs include many of the fundamental verbal, vocal, and body language skills of communication, such as speaking at a reasonable rate of speed, making eye contact with the entire group, and speaking with animation. Initial group exercises, however, may address only one of these skills; more complex interaction exercises often are deferred to later sessions after preliminary competence is demonstrated. An example of a level 1 or 2 Psychosocial Group exercise could be one to train suitable voice volume. The exercise would involve members taking turns giving brief presentations on topics such as: "Who is my favorite actor and why?" or "How do I get from home to here and how long does it take?" while attempting to raise or lower voice level.

After each presentation, other group members give feedback to the presenter, with the group leader providing additional structure in the form of prompts, modeling, examples, and feedback, as necessary. In later sessions of level 1 groups or early sessions of level 2 groups, depending upon the competence and potential of the members, more recreational goals (such as planning an outing for oneself) or interactive goals (e.g., initiating conversation, listening to and summarizing conversation, giving feedback) are attempted.

Level 1 and 2 groups also have curricula that address the important social skill of being able to give and receive positive feedback and suggestions for improvement. Treatment interventions in groups of individuals with greater impairment are very concrete. For instance, when training on giving admiring or appreciative feedback to others, this skill area is practiced across several sessions. The initial exercise may be to generate a list of admiring or appreciative statements (e.g., "Wow, you cooked a great dinner tonight"; "I appreciate you helping me with my knapsack; it was really heavy for me."), and a list of vocal styles and body language that convey sincerity and enthusiasm (e.g., eye contact, smiling, emphasis). Group members then spend several sessions participating in structured two-person role plays in which parts are described (or even scripted) for participants and the goal is to express appreciation or admiration. Following each role play, other group members give feedback regarding the words and phrases used, the vocal style, and the body language of the role play participants. Finally, group members begin structured exercises to express admiration or appreciation of a quality or action in each other (e.g., "I really appreciated it when you smiled at me and said 'Hi' when I joined the group; it made me feel welcome."), with feedback provided by the group and leader.

Level 3. Initial exercises in level 3 Psychosocial Groups include presentations on the following topics: "How am I the same now as I was before my injury (stroke, etc.), and how am I different?" "How has my social life changed since my injury (stroke, etc.), and how is it the same?" Topics are deliberately designed to emphasize both continuity and change in group members, in order to enhance their awareness of how they are the same as or different from the way they used to be. They also help the person combat catastrophic reactions and assist in verbalizing regrets and complaints that will help them formulate individual goals within the group.

Later level 3 group exercises typically use role plays constructed with two or three members as participants. Each member is assigned a role designed to address an individual social skills goal. For example, one member (goal = being inquisitive and keeping conversation flowing) interviews another member (goal = disclosing personal likes/dislikes with greater specificity and confidence) about an interest in jazz. A third group member (goal = giving opinions with less sarcasm) is appointed the role of "feedback-giver." Following the role play this group member evaluates each role player's success in working on his or her goal. Then the feedback-giver is given feedback by other group members and the group leader(s).

Discussion topics in the psychosocial exercise/discussion section are either preplanned and introduced by the leader(s) (e.g., "How do I cope with a rehabilitation therapist I do not like?"), or are developed from a topic brought up by a group member during "Announcements" into a role play situation or discussion. Even in using this more "unstructured" type of exercise, the emphasis is upon participants practicing behaviors to meet individual goals as group members discuss and interact.

SELF-REGULATION GROUPS

Problems in Self-Regulation

The NPS Self-Regulation Groups (SRGs) were initially developed as part of a federally funded grant addressing problem solving in persons with brain injury.[1] For participants in these groups, problems in affective and behavioral regulation are conceptualized as a stumbling block to effective problem solving in that unmodulated emotional responses preclude careful consideration of options or effective implementation of solutions. Unchecked emotional reactions include both "external" loss of control, such as shouting or physical violence, and "internal" reactions, such as a feeling of flooding or mental paralysis, described by one patient as, "My mind goes into a Fifth Avenue traffic jam." Difficulty with affective and behavioral regulation is common in persons with brain injury as a result of a confluence of factors including cognitive deficits (e.g., difficulty processing complex environmental stimuli, difficulty keeping in mind a larger perspective or taking the perspective of another person, all-or-nothing thinking), loss of emotional control (e.g., "short fuse," lability, disproportionate reactions, disinhibition), psychological effects of trauma (e.g., depression, anxiety, increased startle response, poor sleep), and physiological effects of brain injury such as increased fatigue and increased vulnerability and reactivity to environmental stimulation.

These factors interact in a variety of ways, both with each other and with premorbid personality disposition. For example, persons with a preinjury tendency toward a depressive cognitive style may be particularly vulnerable to "all-or-nothing"

[1] The development of these groups was supported in part by NIH grant # 1 RO1 HD 32943-01A1, Leonard Diller, Principal Investigator.

comparisons with premorbid functioning, leading to an increased propensity for disparaging self-statements and catastrophic emotional reactions.

The SRGs are designed to assist individuals with brain injury to become aware of their patterns of difficulties with self-regulation, and to develop ways to recover from and compensate for these difficulties by developing distance and perspective from emotional reactions and increasing the ability to maintain cognitive control over reactions and behaviors.

Structure of Self-Regulation Groups

Selection for SRGs is predicated upon a moderate degree of competence in attention-concentration, awareness of assets and deficits, notetaking, ability to give and receive feedback, and social–emotional skill. However, despite a relatively high level of social and cognitive competence, a structured format is employed that includes the use of a prepared agenda, in-session notetaking, and methods of tracking progress, all crucial to contain and focus discussion and facilitate retention and integration of learned material.

The SRGs are conducted in either a 2-hour session once weekly, or two 1-hour weekly sessions for an 8- to 12-week period, and to follow a protocol of topic-focused modules. The objectives of the modules are: (1) to increase awareness of breakdowns in emotional self-regulation; (2) to analyze each person's pattern of self-regulation difficulties in terms of the relative contributions of (a) processes of disinhibition and loss of emotional control; (b) environmental and physiological factors that increase vulnerability to the above; and (c) disparaging self-talk resulting from unfavorable comparisons with premorbid functioning; (3) to increase awareness and effectiveness of existing strategies for regulating emotions and managing the effects of the three processes listed above; (4) to learn new regulation strategies; (5) to increase awareness of conditions under which breakdowns in emotional self-regulation are likely to occur, anticipate potentially problematic situations, and plan accordingly; and (6) to increase confidence in the capacity for emotional self-management.

Modules and Exercises

Exercises during the course of SRGs have been divided into
modules. In the first module, the concept of self-regulation
is introduced and defined. Examples of breakdowns in self-
regulation are then elicited from group members. The group
leaders use one of the situations provided by members to intro-
duce the method of analyzing the breakdowns. A structured
worksheet is employed, on which group members record specific elements of the process by which breakdowns in self-regulation occur, including probable situations, people, and
internal stressors (illness, lack of sleep, etc.) that trigger the
overly emotional reaction; the initial reaction of the group
member (feelings, thoughts, behaviors, and physical sensations); and the earliest physical, behavioral, and emotional
signs of the reaction sequence occurring. In later sessions of
module 1, group members are taught to analyze their own
breakdowns on the worksheets. Eventually they are given homework involving continued use of the worksheet between sessions to refine awareness of patterns of vulnerability and
response, as well as to begin to become aware of times when the
resolution of the self-regulation situation is more successful.

Successful strategies become the focus of the second module, as each group member participates in a "solution focused"
interview (de Shazer, 1985; de Shazer et al., 1986) about improvements in functioning that already have occurred, strategies or conditions which have contributed to those
improvements, and coping strategies for problems that have
not shown improvement. As a result of this interview, group
members learn that not all of their methods of managing emotional expression are failures, thus counteracting the "all-or-
nothing" mental set. In addition, participants learn to distinguish and appreciate their existing strategies that are successful
or partially successful and to utilize such successes as a basis
for developing a more consistent and deliberate approach to
difficulties with self-regulation.

Once group members have both a general sense of their
pattern of difficulties with self-regulation and some beginning
ideas of strategies that may be helpful, role-play exercises are

introduced in module 3. Role plays use both hypothetical situations generated by the group leader(s) and personal examples of loss of self-regulation brought in by group members as part of an ongoing "homework" assignment. One group member enacts the problem situation, using other members as the "supporting cast." After the initial depiction of the situation, all group members brainstorm alternative ways of responding to and managing the situation. These alternatives are then enacted by the "actors," with breaks in the action to evaluate effectiveness and assess the impact of behavioral changes on internal experience. The beginnings of a list of coping strategies is generated by the group in module 3. Group members use it to suggest alternate behaviors to the actors in the role plays. By processing the action in the role play and postulating other options from the list, members become more competent at analyzing their own behaviors. The competence is reinforced by requiring that group members use between session worksheets to track their self-regulation patterns and the successful implementation of new strategies.

The sequence described above (increase awareness of problems and helpful strategies, brainstorm and role play alternative strategies, implement strategies, and report back) is repeated with a more refined focus on specific problems with: (1) emotional disinhibition (module 4); (2) vulnerability to the effects of environmental and physiological conditions (such as overscheduling combined with excessive fatigue) (module 5); and (3) disparaging self-talk resulting from unfavorable comparisons with premorbid functioning that results in catastrophic reactions or emotional shut-down (module 6).

In the final module of the group (module 7), lists of strategies addressing problems in each of the three focus areas are further detailed and then distributed to each group member. Problems of emotional disinhibition are addressed by a variety of strategies. The early "signals" of reaction patterns are identified (e.g., internal cues or reactions from others indicative of overstepping interpersonal bounds). Members learn to interrupt the pattern by calling for or taking a break in the action (e.g., using calming self-talk, taking deep breaths, counting to 10, tabling the discussion of a provocative situation by politely leaving the scene). These techniques allow the individual to shut down emotional processing temporarily in order to stop escalation of emotional reactivity (e.g., "This is a very important topic, but I just can't think about it clearly right now—let's pick this up later").

Problems related to increased vulnerability to environmental and physiological conditions are addressed by first identifying problematic conditions (e.g., too much activity scheduled for one day; overstimulating environments such crowds or noise; touchy topics of discussion among family members or friends; challenges to one's performance in a work context in light of disability; injury-related symptoms such as fatigue, headaches, and dizziness). Strategies for coping with such vulnerabilities include altering expectations about one's capacity to manage energy and time demands (e.g., reducing frequency of visits with difficult family members, learning to shop for groceries during quiet hours to avoid overstimulation). In addition, such methods are employed as letting others know about limitations, and asking for alterations in conditions which might make the environment more conducive to effective functioning. For example, an important meeting might be scheduled to allow for breaks to accommodate reduced endurance.

Finally, strategies for addressing disparaging self-talk include noticing, analyzing, and replacing negative and self-defeating internal dialogue or self-statements (Burns, 1980). Disparaging self-statements are supplanted with positive, self-enhancing self-statements; "all-or-nothing" thinking with "shades of gray," and comparisons between now and "how I was before the injury" to comparisons between now and "how I was just after I was injured." For example, a person who tells herself that "I can't think as quickly as I used to, so I'm really worthless and useless" practices telling herself instead that, "Even though I can't do things like I used to, I still have something to contribute."

Group members leave the SRG with a printed copy of their group's "Group-Generated Strategies for Self-Regulation." As nearly all the strategies in the list are generated in discussion with group members, the use of a written "official" document serves as a powerful boost to confidence in one's ongoing ability to notice, analyze, and address continuing problems that may emerge. The list also provides the brain injured individual with a tangible reminder of the newly learned skills and a bridge between the group and everyday life.

ANGER MANAGEMENT GROUPS[2]

Problems in Anger Management

Anger Management Groups (AMGs) were designed in response to family and staff reports of marked difficulties with temper control exhibited by some individuals treated on the NPS, e.g., episodes of intense emotionality, shouting, or verbal or physical aggression. The AMGs address specific problems of anger management that are more severe than those targeted in the Self-Regulation Groups. Such difficulties are frequent in the clinical experience of therapists treating patients with acquired brain injury, especially those with underlying cognitive problems associated with injury to the frontal lobes (Mateer & Williams, 1991).

The AMGs are similar to Self-Regulation Groups in that their purpose is to increase cognitive control over emotional processes, but differ in that they are open to persons with a lower level of basic skill and cognitive competence, and have a more specialized focus on emotional and behavioral control of anger. Episodes of loss of anger control are related to the same brain injury-related factors as those interfering with emotional self-regulation (e.g., emotional disinhibition, cognitive impairments such as reduced tolerance for environmental stimulation, loss of ability to maintain a larger perspective or take the perspective of another person, reduced stamina). Such episodes are compounded by other factors including reduced cognitive ability (either postinjury or premorbid) and lower premorbid self-regulation skills related to personality or environmental learning.

---

[2] Anger Management Groups were developed and conducted by Dvorah Simon, Ph.D., Leo J. Shea, III, Ph.D., & Edward Barnowski, Ph.D.

Structure and Content of Anger Management Groups

The AMGs are similar in content to Self-Regulation Groups with some modifications based upon differences in the populations, as described above. The basic format of the Anger Management Group is the same as for all NPS groups, using agendas, structured exercises, notetaking, and homework. Change is implemented by means of discussion, solution-focused interviewing, role plays, and structured worksheets to elicit greater awareness and utilization of effective coping strategies. To accommodate the lower levels of cognitive competence of members of the AMG, the group proceeds at a slower pace, with more concrete discussions, more repetition, and emphasis on careful notetaking. Key points are written on a blackboard by the group leader, and the group leader(s) distribute(s) printed copies of notes from the previous session.

In addition to differences in cognitive competence, many AMG members differ from members of a typical Self-Regulation Group (for whom learning emotional self-regulation often entails recovery of previous social skills) in that they report a greater premorbid tolerance for their own aggressive behaviors. For example, some members, coming from a "street" culture, have argued that unless they can demonstrate the ability to "defend oneself" when insulted, they will be vulnerable to abuse. Others in this group display what appears to be a lifelong personality style of "not taking bulls——t" from anyone. Despite an outwardly tough stance, however, AMG members are often quite sensitive about perceived insults to their self-worth. Issues of self-worth are compounded by deficits in abstract reasoning that lead to an all-or-nothing, black-or-white thinking style, e.g., "If I have a deficit, then I am totally defective."

To address these concerns, the structure of the group is modified somewhat from the SRG to include a preliminary component in which the philosophy of response to insult is examined. To the polarity of passivity versus aggression in the face of insult or frustration is added the option of healthy assertion. Thus the AMG is more psychoeducational in tone than is the SRG. In addition, consequences of uncontrolled anger-based behaviors are explored in a nonjudgmental manner. For example, in answer to the question, "Why is hitting someone not always the best idea?" group members might respond, not with an abstract concept about sublimation being preferable to actions that might harm others, but with the idea that, if caught, such behaviors could lead to undesirable consequences. Group leaders model a respectful tone by accepting such reasoning with gentle suggestions of alternative ways of looking at things, but offer no argument or judgment.

Once the concept of the advisability of alternatives to aggression is established, solution-focused interviewing, worksheets, and role plays are used with a special focus on eliciting strategies of self-calming. Each group member develops a personal list of effective strategies, such as "listening to music when upset" or "thinking about my goals and how what I do might get me there." Issues of self-worth are addressed by paying even more attention than usual to acknowledging group members' contributions and to structuring opportunities for group members to give each other statements of appreciation and support. Group members' self-calming strategies lists are repeatedly reviewed and praised.

The final segment of the group involves review and discussion of anger incidents in the group members' lives. As in the SRG, group members brainstorm and role play alternative strategies for handling the described event, relying on their personal lists for suggestions. Group members reporting successful application of strategies receive positive feedback and support.

SUMMARY/CONCLUSIONS

We have discussed the use of group psychotherapeutic treatment with a brain injured population. The three types of groups described do not exhaust the possibilities for use of this treatment format. Other groups can be conceptualized dealing with specific psychosocial problem areas, e.g., social problems at home or in the work setting, difficulties with social project planning, role changes in the family, and philosophical or spiritual questions about self-concept following the injury.

The many well-known benefits of group treatment apply as well to this population. The important principle in planning such groups is that due to the neuropsychological effects associated with the brain injury, and the consequent problems with psychological adaptation and social skills, these benefits do not occur without explicit planning of group content and format and guidance from the group leader. Groups for individuals with brain injury must be designed to elicit successful group participation and generalization of group gains. With such structure, the therapeutic process for individuals with brain injury can take useful and meaningful form.

REFERENCES

Ben-Yishay, Y., & Diller, L. (1981). Rehabilitation of cognitive and perceptual deficits in people with traumatic brain damage. *International Journal of Rehabilitation Research, 4,* 208–210.

Ben-Yishay, Y., Diller, L., Gerstman, L., & Garden, W. (1970). Relationship between initial competence and ability to profit from cues in brain damaged individuals. *Journal of Abnormal Psychology, 78,* 17–25.

Burns, D. D. (1980). *Feeling good: The new mood therapy.* New York: Morrow.

Deaton, A. V. (1991). Group interventions for cognitive rehabilitation: Increasing the challenges. In J. S. Kreutzer & P. H. Wehman (Eds.), *Cognitive rehabilitation for persons with traumatic brain injury: A functional approach* (pp. 201–214). Baltimore: Paul Brooks.

de Shazer, S. (1985). *Keys to solution in brief therapy.* New York: Norton.

de Shazer, S., Berg, I. K., Lipchik, E., Nunnaly, E., Molnar, A., Gingrich, W., & Weiner-Davis, M. (1986). Brief therapy: Focused solution development. *Family Process, 25,* 207–222.

Langer, K. G. (1992). Psychotherapy with the neuropsychologically-impaired adult. *American Journal of Psychotherapy, 46,* 620–639.

Lewis, L., & Rosenberg, S. J. (1990). Psychoanalytic psychotherapy with brain-injured adult psychiatric patients. *Journal of Nervous and Mental Disease, 178,* 69–77.

Mateer, C. A., & Williams, D. (1991). Management of psychosocial and behavior problems in cognitive rehabilitation. In J. S. Kreutzer & P. H. Wehman (Eds.), *Cognitive rehabilitation for persons with traumatic brain injury: A functional approach* (pp. 117–126). Baltimore: Paul Brooks.

Miller, L. (1993). *Psychotherapy of the brain-injured patient: Reclaiming the shattered self.* New York: Norton.

Prigatano, G. P., Fordyce, D. J., Zeiner, H. K., Roueche, F. R., Pepping, M., & Wood, B. C. (Eds.). (1986). *Neuropsychological rehabilitation after brain injury.* Baltimore: Johns Hopkins University Press.

Prigatano, G. P., & Schacter, D. L. (1991). *Awareness of deficit after brain injury: Clinical and theoretical issues.* New York: Oxford University Press.

Sherr, R. L., & Langenbahn, D. M. (1992). An approach to large-scale outpatient neuropsychological rehabilitation. *Neuropsychology, 6,* 417–426.

Weiner, I. B. (1966). *Psychodiagnosis in schizophrenia.* New York: Wiley.

Yalom, I. D. (1985). *The theory and practice of group psychotherapy* (3rd ed.). New York: Basic Books.

10.

Psychotherapeutic Issues in Treating Family Members

Frank J. Padrone, Ph.D.

Advances in medical technology have led to increased survival from brain injury due either to traumatic brain injury (TBI), cerebral vascular accident (stroke), or surgical interventions, such as those for brain tumor.

Rehabilitation services for people with neuropsychological disabilities have been steadily increasing over the past few decades. Sophisticated neuropsychological diagnosis and treatment are now commonplace in rehabilitation (Diller, 1987). The process of psychological adjustment to physical disability has been well described by Janis and Leventhal (1965), Langer (1994), and McDaniel (1976), as have the approaches to family therapy directed at the adjustment process of the family group with a member who has a physical disability (Parry & Young, 1978; Whiting, Terry, & Strom-Henrikson, 1984).

The increased survival rate amongst the TBI/stroke population has led to an escalation in the number of family members who suffer stress as a result. Many rehabilitation professionals feel that psychological intervention with family members is essential (Prigatano, 1987). Since this need is not often fulfilled, many family members are referred increasingly outside the rehabilitation system for individual psychotherapy to help them cope with the situation.

The stress experienced by the family in response to physical disability with neuropsychological impairment may be somewhat different from that experienced in response to a disability without a neuropsychological component. Although stress subsequent to loss, family disruption, dependence, and practical concerns are similar, the challenge to cope with consequences of neuropsychological impairment presents relatively unique considerations. The possibility of altered personality and impaired cognitive skills is not so readily understood by most people as are the physical changes that pose a challenge to adjustment. Such characteristics need to be addressed in any comprehensive treatment regimen.

DISABILITY AND THE FAMILY

Family members struggle with issues at once similar to and different from those of the person with the disability. The focus here is on issues to be considered when a relative of a person with a neuropsychological impairment is seen in psychotherapy with the goal of helping them to cope better with the stress. The age of the person with the disability most probably assumes a bimodal distribution, since the disabilities represented form two major groups: Traumatic brain injury occurs primarily below age 35 (Williamson, Scott, & Adams, 1996), and stroke (CVA) occurs primarily over age 65, although 20% are below age 65 (Binder, Howieson, & Coull, 1987).

The family member as patient may present for treatment with feelings of confusion, depression, anxiety, guilt, and/or desperation. If the onset of the disability has been recent, he or she may be feeling overwhelmed and may be in crisis. Family members in need of treatment may not have had the opportunity or necessary support to deal with their own reactions, since the focus of attention has been primarily on the person who suffered the disability. By necessity the family members have been the responsible ones. Often having been encouraged to become a member of the rehabilitation team, the family member has shouldered a disproportionate share of the burden. The natural reaction of denial may foster this state in which the family member has not yet processed the event emotionally.

The adjustment process for those who suffer traumatic disabilities includes familiar stages (McDaniel, 1976). Reactions to major losses, such as those occurring with disability, are similar to those posited by Kübler-Ross (1970) in her work on the knowledge of one's own impending death. Denial, anger, depression, and adjustment are the reactions that are now familiar in the field. It may be said that family members experience a similar loss process, the intensity of which is commensurate with the relative meaning of the disability for them and the relationship to the person with the disability (Padrone, 1994).

Whether the therapeutic intervention targets the individual family member, the entire family, or some subunit, familiarity with family therapy concepts will be useful in the work with family members of those with disabilities. In family systems therapy the focus of treatment is the family unit rather than the individual. It is necessary for this unit to accommodate to major changes in the life cycle for optimal functioning (Minuchin, 1974). When changes, such as a birth, a death, or a disability occur, adaptation within the family unit is required. The balance within the family system has been altered by a tragedy with which the family and its individual members must contend.

The structural analytic approach to family therapy utilizes an individual and systems perspective (Kantor, 1983) that focuses on perceptions held by individuals and the family group in the present and past. This approach advocates that members have developed views of inner and outer reality that comprise their anticipations and expectations of others, and enhance communication. These views provide the foundation for intimacy, since through them the members can share a common view of reality. Such views when applied to the self in connection to others are the ones we hold about relationships. If some event leads to conflict between the views of any two people, an impediment to family growth develops, so that the family may become blocked in the adaptation process (Munro, 1985). The

process of adjustment may be blocked by a number of considerations, such as personality characteristics or situational factors.
For example, those who tend to cope by blaming others, or
even themselves, may become stuck in the process, while issues
such as quality of the premorbid relationship, the extent of
dependence, or frustrations with helping organizations in the
community also may be an impediment. In some instances the
disability may serve as a scapegoat, when other problems exist
in the relationship which would produce significant anxiety if
they were to be addressed.

Using a systems perspective Turnbull and Turnbull (1990)
examine the impact of disability on the family by considering
(1) the family; (2) the disability; (3) individuals within the family; and (4) the network of relationships (subsystems) that exist
within the family. For example, the extent of disability and the
coping styles of family members influence both the experience
of the disability and the adjustment process. All of the relationships within the family will be impacted by the disability. The
integration of this change will be influenced by the extent to
which the family does not become chaotic in its function, but
is flexible, and does not rigidly hold on to former ways of managing. If the family can remain cohesive and not become en-
meshed in the details of the disability, while trying to support
the person with the disability, the probability of a satisfactory
adjustment is enhanced. Family values and cultures are also
seen to influence adjustment. For example, cultural differences
in attitude toward disability, changing family roles, or issues
regarding dependence have significant impact on adjustment.

The general conceptualizations regarding disability, family
systems, and interventions can be useful only when considering
the specific context of the sequelae of brain injury. Neuropsychological impairments present challenges to adjustment, not
only because they are often major losses with which the family
must cope, but also by their very nature. The losses are not so
easily understood as are physical losses. For example, it takes a
relatively short time for a family member to realize many of
the physical limitations consequent to a T10 paraplegia or
hemiplegia with the aid of brief instruction and imagination.
The same cannot be said for the consequences of a moderate

attention deficit or a significant visual field neglect. In addition, cognitive and personality changes are experienced as yielding a different person, which is not the case in a T10 paraplegia. Just as adjustment to physical changes is influenced by different cultural systems and personal psychological issues, so too is adjustment to neuropsychological changes.

THE PATIENT

Since psychotherapy in some form is increasingly recommended for relatives of people with disability secondary to brain injury, especially following TBI (Prigatano, 1987), and also after stroke (Binder et al., 1987), the identification of the patient and the locus of treatment is less predictable. Regardless, many of the ongoing processes described above are brought into treatment. The patient may be struggling to cope with the realization of such significant impairments in their loved one that he or she is overwhelmed, especially if there is a lack of understanding of the neuropsychological elements. He or she may be attempting to deal with the disruptive impact of the disability on the relationship, current family functioning, issues regarding extended family, lack of resources, and integration with extended family, friends, and the community. If the patient is also the caregiver, there are additional sources of stress.

Given the enormity of the above stressors, the patient's emotional reactions nonetheless can be easily overlooked until they have become quite intense. If the patient is referred for treatment while in the initial throes of distress, the therapeutic management of reactions to such trauma is not an unusual task for the therapist. The patient may be intensely experiencing some stage of the coping process, e.g., denial, anger, or grieving. Although there is a danger in becoming absorbed in the practical aspects of the disability and its consequences, knowledge of the neuropsychological impairment is necessary for therapist and patient. In the process of psychotherapy it is not unusual for a patient to educate the therapist about some area of experience with which the therapist has little familiarity. In this situation, however, the patient is in the process of learning the information not only for practical reasons, but also to aid in emotional adjustment. The realization that a spouse no longer remembers key events shared in the past, or is having difficulty concentrating sufficiently to carry on more than a brief conversation, is a major loss to be processed. Within the context of the patient's ability to cope, the therapist may need to advocate for education, since resistance to such information may often represent denial of painful realities. Since the possibility exists that the patient's more intense feelings may have been labeled as inappropriate in quality or degree by others, support for such feelings may be indicated. For example, there may have been open or subtle disapproval of the patient's angry feelings, so that support for such a reaction while monitoring its intensity may be necessary. In time, however, the use of anger as a defense against the more painful feelings of grieving may also need to be explored.

In the early phase of treatment the patient may experience considerable guilt. It may be difficult to tolerate the not uncommon wish to flee from stress, responsibilities, and the feelings of anger or disgust over major physical changes. The experience of such repressed feelings can produce considerable anxiety or conflict, which may be relieved only when the patient has been able to make a distinction between the disability per se and the person with it. For example, one may be angry about another's behavior and the injury that has caused it, without being angry at the person with the disability. In like manner, one may wish to be free of the responsibilities, but not necessarily the person associated with them.

Although "acceptance" of the disability (Kübler-Ross, 1970) is often seen as an important goal of treatment (Vargo, 1979), the connotation that the person somehow has agreed to this terrible state of affairs leads to resentment and resistance in many. The advice to "accept reality" during the struggle for adjustment may have an unfortunate connotation (Padrone, 1994). In order to deal with such resistance it may be helpful to indicate that painful realities can be acknowledged. They can be integrated into the psyche and permitted to take their place in reality without one having to like them.

Feelings of shame may develop in reaction to having a family member who is disabled and different. Such feelings, when coupled with the inability of the person with the disability to fully participate socially, may lead to isolation. The restriction or elimination of many family social events and activities (Lezak, 1988) can lead to resentment and alienation.

THE TREATMENT

Treatment interventions with such patients should be multidimensional. Rosenthal (1984) has recommended a four-part program with families of those with brain injury that includes education, counseling, therapy, and support groups. Extent of family involvement is dependent on variations in disability and in family function. It has been our experience that a similar four-layered approach is often indicated: education, family intervention, direct psychotherapy for a family member(s), and referral to community resources, such as a support group.

The educational layer evolves from the fact that in addition to the physical and emotional components of the disability, neuropsychological changes are not easily comprehended. Families may benefit from information provided by publications such as *Stroke: Why Do They Behave That Way?* (Fowler & Fordyce, 1974).

Without information regarding the consequences of brain injury the family may attempt to explain their loved one's behavior in terms with which they are familiar that can be primarily physical, psychological, or even moralistic. In addition to the conflict that usually arises from such misinterpretations, the patient is deprived of the opportunity for the use of better management strategies, but also of the necessary emotional processing of a loss. Brief outlines of the possible changes following brain injury may be presented to the family member(s) with some discussion of the factors that are relevant for them.

When necessary education is not provided, family members can fall victim to misinterpretations similar to those that follow:

Impairment in arousal may be seen as depression or lack of motivation.

Impairment of attention may be labeled as disinterest, inconsiderateness, or willfulness.

Memory impairments may be misinterpreted as resistance, denial, or confusion.

Impulsivity may be seen as merely being "in a hurry" or stubbornly doing it their way.

Diminished ability to initiate may be seen as depression, dependence, or laziness.

Family members often believe that those with *aphasia* understand more than they actually do, and when the impairment is misinterpreted, they are thought to be confused, disoriented, or uncooperative and hostile.

The misreading of an *impaired ability to abstract* may be seen as stubbornness, rather than rigidity of thought, or procrastination rather than the inability to plan ahead.

Problems due to *perceptual losses* may be interpreted as poor motivation or confusion and disorientation.

A change in the ability to *express and control affect* may be misinterpreted as solely depression or willfulness.

A *lack of awareness* of disability may be misinterpreted as solely due to emotionally based denial, when in fact neurological and neuropsychological factors may be at work.

Family Intervention

Lezak (1986) suggests that discussions should be held with family members concerning the following:

1. Feelings of anger, frustration, and sorrow should be identified as natural and to be expected.
2. Caretakers must not minimize their own needs.
3. Caretakers should rely on their own conscience and judgment to deal with conflicts.
4. Role changes that occur may be distressing to everyone.

5. Family members should avoid the use of a guilt model for not doing more, but rather weigh all aspects of the situation, including the eventual price to be paid if other decisions are made.

6. When the welfare of dependent children is at stake, the conflict arising from divided loyalties should be acknowledged and responsibilities should be prioritized.

Family intervention can utilize an educational and counseling approach, or include active family therapy.

A number of factors need to be considered in the third layer, psychotherapy with these patients including initiation of therapy; severity of disability; onset issues; stage of rehabilitation; relationship to the disabled; life stage; meaning of disability; preexisting relationship; dynamics of relationship; and countertransference.

Initiation of Therapy

Although some rehabilitation programs provide routine intervention for all families of both head injury and stroke patients, a significant portion do not. In the former group families may be seen for education and some counseling, and in the latter group such interventions are provided only when family members are referred for psychotherapy after significant distress is perceived. Even where education and counseling may be routine, the focus appears to be on the person with the disability, and not on the difficulties of the family member, as is usually the context for individual psychotherapy. In this regard the patient may perceive the atmosphere to be one in which the person with the disability should be the "real patient," and he or she is not the focus of treatment. Such a perception may contribute to an experience in which the therapist is perceived as having split loyalties or "an agenda," as in our experience many family members have commented.

Although unfortunately at times this perception may be accurate, it also can reflect feelings of guilt or resistance in the family member, when he or she experiences their own treatment as a shift in focus of attention from the person with the disability. The patient can feel undeserving of such attention, especially since he or she remains unscathed.

Attention to the ordeal of the family member also can lead to feelings of anxiety. Such anxiety can stem from a growing awareness of suppressed, ambivalent feelings regarding the situation, the disability, and the person with the disability. For example, the disability may have resulted from a life-threatening situation, leading to thoughts as to whether the person with the disability might have been better off if he or she had not survived. Such thoughts are not uncommon, as are the concomitant feelings of guilt and anger that often underlie them.

The severity of disability both physically and neuropsychologically is directly proportionate to the extent of loss and change in the life of the family member. Physical dependence and cognitive dependence clearly produce different effects which are not identical for different families or even family members. In the domain of everyday labor, who takes out the trash, does the cooking and shopping, balances the checkbook, provides child care, and produces the bulk of family income may be differentially impacted contingent on the preexisting distribution of these responsibilities.

Lezak (1988) suggests that there is a direct correlation between the extent of neuropsychological deficits and the impact on family members, which can be crushing to a relationship. The stress from changes in roles, finances, and social status are exacerbated by the common social isolation and loss of emotional supports to these families.

It has been suggested that the presence of any of the following three factors places families at high risk in terms of eventual adjustment: (1) premorbid history of significant family problems, such as marital conflict or alcoholism; (2) an inordinately long period of denial; or (3) persistent, severe cognitive or physical impairments (Rosenthal, 1984).

Contingent on severity of disability the effect on social lives can range from totally destroyed to minimally changed. Levels of companionship, partnership, and intimacy can also be impacted in varying degrees. Once again premorbid lifestyles and values must be taken into account when considering the degree of loss.

There can be a sudden increase in the workload, leading to fatigue and resentment. Family members may become caretakers and experience themselves in a parental role, while the person with the disability becomes infantilized. Significant physical or cognitive dependence can lead patients to consider the person with the disability as inferior. Such a perception is supported by a comparative value system in societies (Dembo, Leviton, & Wright, 1956), rather than a system that values people's assets, regardless of how they measure up to others.

As noted earlier, if the family has not been educated regarding neuropsychological changes, they can misinterpret such changes or their consequences, leading to conflict and interminable frustration. Personality changes are common with significant brain injury, especially in TBI, so that the patient can now experience the family member with the disability as no longer the same person. Not only are aspects of the person with the disability lost, leaving patients feeling isolated and abandoned, but they can be replaced by irritability, impulsivity, socially inappropriate behavior, diminished sensitivity to others, and affective disturbances in varying degrees (Prigatano, 1987). Exacerbating the situation is the fact that the person with the disability may not be aware of many of these difficulties.

Issues associated with the **onset of the disability** can influence significantly the adjustment process for the patient. Does the patient hold the person responsible for the disability due to some imprudent action, or does he or she in some way hold him- or herself responsible for the disability? For example, it may have followed a heated argument or the patient may have been driving the car in which the person with the disability was injured. Clearly such issues can influence the patient's feelings and adjustment.

In the early **stage of rehabilitation** the family member may be struggling to cope with the initial crisis, the acute symptoms of neuropsychological impairment, and adjustment reactions to loss, in addition to the distress of the person with the disability. After transition to the outpatient phase of rehabilitation family members may be struggling openly with their own depression and anxiety, while hoping that specific abilities will be recovered. As rehabilitation comes to an end, treatment of the disability is no longer the focus, but the need to live with it is at hand. "The family and the person with the disability are now more on their own dealing with the day-to-day problems of the disability, its chronicity, and its impact on all aspects of life" (Padrone, 1994, p. 201).

Clearly during this period the patient, the person with the disability, and the entire family unit are progressing through a mourning process. It has been suggested by Leber and Jenkins (1996) that since the person with the disability has survived as a new and different individual, the ritual is incomplete. The people involved are mourning abilities and qualities of a person, while adjusting to a person who behaves differently.

The **relationship to the disabled** defines many of the changes with which the patient will contend. A *spouse, child, parent,* or *sibling* will be coping with different issues.

The *spouse* of the person with the disability has lost much of the partner whom he or she knew. Role changes, with their concomitant threats to ego and value systems are common. Changes in sex lives are also common, including matters of intimacy and privacy, especially if attendant help in the home is required.

A significant percentage of couples report that their sexual activity had ceased following a stroke (Ducharme, 1987). In addition, in TBI there also may be major sexual changes ranging from disinhibition to loss of interest. There are many anecdotal reports and some surveys on sexual activity following neuropsychological changes, but as Lezak suggests (as cited in Leber and Jenkins, 1996) the cognitive and behavioral sequelae of brain injury explain most of the difficulties, even weighing the limitations from the physical changes.

Sexuality is certainly one of the central components in a couple's relationship, and should be a significant part of the treatment. It has been observed in Western cultures that there may be an undue emphasis on the role of sexual intercourse in sexual intimacy and satisfaction (Glass and Padrone, 1978).

Approaches to preserving these aspects of the relationship without sexual intercourse should be explored where indicated. In order to accomplish such goals, the treatment will probably need to include elements of the grieving process to address this important issue. When such issues are openly addressed in the therapy, the patient may be obliged to deal with his or her own sexuality. Ignoring such issues increases the probability of long-term frustrations and a lack of intimacy. It should be noted that there may be a tendency by therapists who are not experienced in this area to omit this important topic.

The patient who is the *parent* may be truly ambivalent in the face of enormous responsibility. There may be resentment regarding the loss of an expected future, and anger if there is a question of imprudent actions contributing to the disability. The reawakening of conflicts from the earlier relationship leads to feelings that are commonly laced with guilt.

The patient who is a *child* of someone with a disability can be affected even more by the previous relationship, including unresolved needs, past grievances, conflicts over role reversals, and the keen awareness of issues of mortality.

The patient who is a *sibling* may be distressed during younger years due to an awakening of issues of vulnerability and possibly survivor guilt. The history of the relationship between siblings can be fertile ground for conflicted feelings, including anger over this family disruption and anxiety regarding future responsibilities.

Although a disability strikes at a **specific period of life,** it does not remain static but is dynamic, since the life stages continue to change (Williams & Kay, 1991). Although the stage of onset may carry with it its own tasks with which it may interact (Turnbull & Turnbull, 1990), there also will be an interaction with all of the remaining stages for each of the family members and the entire family unit.

The **meaning** of the disability significantly influences the effect it has on the patient from two perspectives: (1) the apparent meaning which derives from the obvious practical consequences, e.g., physical dependence, workload, or loss of a companion whom one knew; and (2) the inner or psychological meaning which derives from its psychodynamic influences.

Does the change in the person with the disability present a threat to the patient in ego terms? Are well-developed coping skills or defensive strategies that were used to negotiate life rendered useless, thereby disrupting psychic equilibrium? Very often these are the issues that need to be addressed when treating the patient.

In addition, the disability of the loved one may lead the patient to experience certain inner conflicts, such as exposing repressed personality characteristics, e.g., unresolved dependency issues or exposing personality difficulties, which compromise functioning when challenged by the presence of the disability.

The **preexisting relationship** includes elements that are generally considered assets as well as those considered liabilities. Preexisting conflicts in the relationship can be exacerbated by the new demands and stress imposed by the disability. "Each family . . . has weaknesses that, given a particular triggering event or circumstance, can lead to serious family dysfunction" (Parry and Young, 1978, p. 64). Grievances or dissatisfactions that had been dormant or tolerated can limit the patient's capacity to extend him- or herself during this period, or additional demands can disrupt a previous delicate balance. It may be said that the quality of the relationship between any two people contributes to its ability to withstand stress. Conversely the poorer the relationship the more vulnerable it may be. It is equally important to note the impact that the stress of disability has on the dynamic balance of the relationship.

The balance of the respective psychodynamics of the persons involved, and how that balance is altered by the disability, significantly influences the impact it will have on the relationship (Padrone, 1994). The disability may negate the primary supports of the relationship or it may result in some intolerable conflict either within one of the parties or between them. Clearly if the positive supports of a relationship are removed, the stress of the disability may be more difficult to tolerate. If certain critical ego "needs" that had been supplied in the relationship are now absent, even a relatively mild disability can be disastrous to the relationship, especially if issues of self-esteem are at stake. For example, when characteristics of a partner that have maintained the self-esteem of the other are eliminated by even a mild neuropsychological impairment, the relationship may be in jeopardy.

Although the loss of any ability, such as earning a living or being socially active, is stressful, it appears to be the meaning of that loss at multiple levels that is critical. Not only the practical and emotional consequences need to be examined with the patient, but also the interpersonal, intrapsychic, and system (family) influences may need consideration. The following example may demonstrate more clearly this multidimensional perspective:

> [I]f a member of a couple is more dependent as a result of a (neuropsychological) disability . . . for the able-bodied person (patient) there is probably more work at a practical level, which (can be) . . . disruptive and require burdensome responsibility.
>
> Personally, (the patient) will need to experience the grieving process regarding all areas of living impacted by this loss, e.g., the patient's image of the partner with the disability and what he or she had been able to do, the inability to attend certain functions together (inaccessibility), the inability to dance or make love. . . .
>
> Interpersonally, role reversals . . . can be burdensome, stressful, (and) produce conflict due to a clash with personal values or cultural beliefs. . . . Within the family unit changes in responsibilities and style of managing, e.g., disciplining young children will have ripple effects. . . .
>
> Intrapsychically if a concealed dependence on the part of the patient can no longer be satisfied . . . not only is the frustration and . . . angry depression a problem, but the experience . . . of the repressed need, (can) result in anxiety and defensive irritability. (Padrone, 1994, p. 203)

The topic of **countertransference** is addressed in detail in another chapter, so that the following comments are limited to those issues that are relevant to the treatment of family members of those with neuropsychological impairment. Although countertransference in psychotherapy is commonly addressed in the training of dynamic psychotherapists, the effect on the therapist of the emotionally laden issues of mortality, physical and neuropsychological disability, and sexuality and disability are not commonly considered. Furthermore, given the value that is probably placed on cognitive function by those who have pursued graduate education, the area of neuropsychological impairment can be especially vulnerable to unexplored countertransferential reactions.

When treating a family member within the rehabilitation system, there is the possibility of identification by the therapist with the needs of the person with the disability, who may be seen as the "primary patient" in that setting. Such identification limits choices for the family member, and often limits a full exploration of the problems. Conversely, when a family member is treated outside of the rehabilitation system, the unrecognized countertransference to neuropsychological disability may have the opposite effect, causing the psychotherapist to align with the patient's anxiety, and limit the exploration of the dynamic roots of the problem within the patient. Regardless of the setting and source of these often subtle countertransferential reactions, both the patient and the person with the disability are underserved.

The very fact that the patient is struggling to cope with reality-based changes and losses that appear so evident is what makes them vulnerable to easy identification and unrecognized countertransference by the therapist. Lastly, as a more subtle indication of countertransference there may be a tendency to focus on concrete solutions or strategies for the patient, since the "causes" of the problem are seen as physical.

The fourth layer of the approach, *referral to community resources,* can be very useful during and after the outpatient phase of treatment. Groups sponsored by the National Head Injury Association and local Stroke Clubs can offer education, insight, and considerable support.

RECOMMENDATIONS

Since there is an increasing need for treatment of family members of those with neuropsychological disabilities, there is a need for specific training in these areas for those who deliver psychotherapeutic services (Kemp & Mallinckrodt, 1996). Some of the stress-producing content for therapists is quite specific, and produces a high probability for unrecognized countertransference. Hornby and Seligman (1991) point out that even though there has been some effort to provide counseling skills to those working in these areas, access to such training is not readily available. Just as many doctoral level programs in psychology are now providing training in neuropsychology, benefit would derive from more specific training in providing psychotherapeutic services to persons with physical and neuropsychological impairment and their family members.

SUMMARY

The need for individual psychotherapy for family members of persons with neuropsychological disabilities is growing as medical interventions improve and survival rates increase. The family members' grief reactions are one part of the adjustment process. Psychological difficulties that develop are influenced by a number of considerations.

The family member who is the psychotherapy patient is part of a family unit whose balance, functioning, and development have been disrupted. Factors relevant to physical disability, family systems approaches, and psychodynamic theory are influential in the treatment. The severity and type of a relative's disability determine the practical and personal impact for the patient, as does the relationship of the patient to the person with the disability. A spouse, parent, child or sibling will each experience different practical and emotional consequences within the context of his or her stage of life and culture. The circumstances of the onset of the disability, the quality of the relationship, and the psychodynamic balance within each person and within the relationship are important issues to consider.

All of the above affects the meaning of the disability for each family member personally, interpersonally, intrapsychically, and within the family unit. Because of limited experience with these emotionally loaded issues, possibilities for unrecognized countertransference are significant. Recommendation is made for increased exposure to the area of neuropsychological disability in the training of psychotherapists.

REFERENCES

Binder, L. M., Howieson, D., & Coull, B. M. (1987). Stroke: Causes and consequences. In B. Caplan (Ed.), *Rehabilitation psychology desk reference* (pp. 65–99). Rockland, MD: Aspen.

Dembo, T., Leviton, G. L., & Wright, B. A. (1956). Adjustment to misfortune—A problem of social psychological rehabilitation. *Artificial Limbs, 3,* 4–62.

Diller, L. (1987). Neuropsychological rehabilitation. In M. Meier, A. Benton, & L. Diller (Eds.), *Neuropsychological rehabilitation* (pp. 1–17). New York: Guilford.

Ducharme, S. (1987). Sexuality and physical disability. In B. Caplan (Ed.), *Rehabilitation psychology desk reference* (pp. 419–435). Rockland, MD: Aspen.

Fowler, S. R., & Fordyce, W. E. (1974). *Stroke: Why do they behave that way?* WA: Washington State Heart Association.

Glass, D. D., & Padrone, F. J. (1978). Sexual adjustment in the handicapped. *Journal of Rehabilitation, 44,* 43–47.

Hornby, G., & Seligman, M. (1991). Disability and the family: Current status and future developments. *Counseling Psychology Quarterly, 4,* 267–271.

Janis, F. L., & Leventhal, H. (1965). Psychological aspects of physical illness and hospital care. In B. B. Wolman (Ed.), *Handbook of clinical psychology* (pp. 1360–1377). New York: McGraw-Hill.

Kantor, D. (1983). The structural-analytic approach to the treatment of family developmental crisis. *Family Therapy Collections, 7,* 12–34.

Kemp, N. T., & Mallinckrodt, B. (1996). Impact of professional training on case conceptualization of clients with a disability. *Professional Psychology: Research and Practice, 27,* 378–385.

Kübler-Ross, E. (1970). *On death and dying.* New York: Macmillan.

Langer, K. G. (1994). Depression and denial in psychotherapy of persons with disabilities. *American Journal of Psychotherapy, 48,* 181–194.

Leber, W. R., & Jenkins, M. R. (1996). Psychotherapy with clients who have brain injuries and their families. In R. Adams, O. Parsons, J.

Culbertson, & S. Nixon (Eds.), *Neuropsychology for clinical practice* (pp. 489–506). Washington, DC: American Psychological Association.

Lezak, M. D. (1986). Psychological implications of traumatic brain injury for the patient's family. *Rehabilitation Psychology, 31,* 241–250.

Lezak, M. D. (1988). Brain damage is a family affair. *Journal of Clinical and Experimental Neuropsychology, 10,* 111–123.

McDaniel, J. W. (1976). *Physical disability and human behavior.* New York: Pergamon.

Minuchin, S. (1974). *Families and family therapy.* Cambridge, MA: Harvard University Press.

Munro, J. D. (1985). Counseling severely dysfunctional families of mentally and physically disabled persons. *Clinical Social Work Journal, 13,* 18–31.

Padrone, F. J. (1994). Psychotherapeutic issues with family members of persons with physical disabilities. *American Journal of Psychotherapy, 48,* 195–207.

Parry, J. K., & Young, A. K. (1978). The family as a system in hospital-based social work. *Health and Social Work, 3,* 54–70.

Prigatano, G. P. (1987). Personality and psychosocial consequences after brain injury. In M. Meier, A. Benton, & L. Diller (Eds.), *Neuropsychological rehabilitation* (pp. 355–378). New York: Guilford.

Rosenthal, M. (1984). Strategies for family intervention. In B. Edelstein & E. Couture (Eds.), *Behavioral approaches to the traumatically brain injured* (pp. 227–246). New York: Plenum.

Turnbull, A. P., & Turnbull, H. R. (1990). *Families, professionals and exceptionality—A special partnership.* Columbus, MD: Charles E. Merrill.

Vargo, J. W. (1979). The disabled wife and mother: Suggested goals for family counseling. *Canadian Counsellor, 13,* 108–111.

Whiting, R. A., Terry, L. L., & Strom-Henrikson, H. (1984). An interactional approach to treating the symptomatic disabled college student. *Family Therapy Collections, 11,* 30–43.

Williams, J. M., & Kay, T. (1991). *Head injury a family matter.* Baltimore: Paul Brooks.

Williamson, D. J., Scott, J. G., & Adams, R. L. (1996). Traumatic brain injury. In R. L. Adams, O. A. Parsons, J. L. Culbertson, & S. J. Nixon (Eds.), *Neuropsychology for clinical practice* (pp. 9–64). Washington, DC: American Psychological Association.

11.

Substance Abuse Interventions for People with Brain Injury

Mary F. Schmidt, Ph.D. and
Allen W. Heinemann, Ph.D.

Each year an estimated 1.9 million people experience traumatic brain injury (Collins, 1990); approximately 80,000 experience continuing, significant disability (National Foundation for Brain Research, 1994). Alcohol and other drug (AOD) abuse is a major risk factor for acquired brain injury. Although alcohol is the primary drug associated with acquired brain injury, the use of other drugs such as benzodiazepines, marijuana, opiates, barbiturates, and amphetamine has also been linked with acquired brain injury (Kreutzer, Wehman, Harris, Burns, & Young, 1991; Boyle, Vella, & Maloney, 1991). Alcohol

Acknowledgments. This work was funded in part by the National Institute of Disability and Rehabilitation Research Demonstration Project (84-133a): H133A10014-93 and the Rehabilitation Services Administration Contract #H128A00002 (Midwest Regional Head Injury Center for Rehabilitation and Prevention) to the Rehabilitation Institute of Chicago. The authors wish to acknowledge the significant contributions of the following coinvestigators of the NIDRR project: Miles Cox, Ph.D., S. Vincent Miranti, Ph.D., Eric Klinger, Ph.D., and Joseph Blount, Ph.D., who adapted Systematic Motivational Counseling at Schwab Rehabilitation Center; Mary Ridgely, C.R.C. and Mervin Langley, Ph.D., who applied Skills-Based Substance Abuse Prevention Counseling within the Wisconsin Vocational Rehabilitation system; and all the people who participated in this project.

use is implicated in 48% of all fatal motor vehicle crashes and upward to 72% of all brain injuries (Kreutzer, Doherty, Harris, & Zasler, 1990; Sparadeo, Strauss, & Barth, 1990; Kreutzer, Wehman et al., 1991). Moreover, alcohol abusers are more likely to be involved in repeat motor vehicle crashes (McLellan et al., 1993) and other traumatic injury-producing events such as falls.

The connection between AOD use and the occurrence of traumatic brain injury has been well established. Corrigan and colleagues (Corrigan, Rust, & Lamb-Hart, 1995) noted that approximately two-thirds of patients admitted to brain injury rehabilitation programs have a history of alcohol or other drug use that can be described as abusive. Among a sample of people interviewed one year after discharge from inpatient rehabilitation for brain injury, at least one half reported resumption of alcohol use (Schmidt & Garvin, 1994). Kreutzer, Witol, and Marwitz (1996) have found that 2 years after injury, alcohol use patterns often return to preinjury levels.

A personal history of alcohol or other drug use has been associated with deterioration of functioning after brain injury (Dunlop, Udvarhelyi, Stedem, & O'Connor, 1991). This may be explained by a number of factors. For example, intoxication may interact with the brain injury itself to increase the resulting cognitive or motor impairments (Kreutzer et al., 1991). People with a history of AOD abuse, especially chronic abuse, may have fewer financial, social, and medical resources including social supports, to facilitate their continued recovery. In addition, the use of substances following acquired brain injury is potentially dangerous when combined with prescription medications and may increase the likelihood of seizures (Murray, 1987). Resumption of substance use following brain injury is associated with continued significant cognitive deficits (Parsons, 1987). Other negative sequelae of substance use after brain injury include increased balance problems, depression, and increased suicide risk (as cited by Langley & Kiley, 1992).

Complicating the picture is the fact that alcohol and other drug use or abuse can cause transient or permanent brain dysfunction. A perusal of the American Psychiatric Association's

Diagnostic and Statistical Manual (4th ed., DSM-IV, 1994) underscores this point. Alcohol and other drug effects can run the behavioral gamut from delirium to dementia. However, there is no reliable way to accurately predict the effect alcohol or other drugs can or will have on a person's cognitive or behavioral functioning; complex biopsychosocial factors are involved in determining the effect that substances have on a person's functioning. In fact, some people acquire neuropsychological dysfunction (e.g., alcoholic dementia) solely through the direct action of substances that can be neurotoxic, rather than through indirect or secondary effects, such as increased risk of traumatic brain injury or nutritional deficits.

Prudence suggests that identification, prevention, and treatment of substance problems should be integral components of rehabilitation, especially given the increasing focus on increasing rehabilitation efficacy and improving outcomes. If approximately two of three participants in brain injury rehabilitation programs are potentially at risk for less than optimal outcome and quality of life secondary to AOD use, brain injury rehabilitation professionals would be wise to incorporate substance use intervention strategies in their rehabilitation programs. However, rehabilitation professionals often lack basic information regarding the identification, assessment, and intervention of substance use problems among clientele (Kiley, Heinemann et al., 1992; Moore, 1992), and few specialized intervention programs are available (Corrigan, Lamb-Hart, & Rust, 1995; Jones, 1992; Schmidt & Garvin, 1994).

Research has shown that substance abuse treatment among the general population has variable outcomes. Relapses among patients who have received formal substance abuse treatment continue at a high rate (Donovan & Chaney, 1985; Marlatt & Gordon, 1985), but is minimized when treatment components meet client expectations. Components of successful treatment include the development of positive alternatives to substance use (Valliant, 1983; Tucker, Vuchinich, & Harris, 1985) and feelings of satisfaction with life (Polich, Armor, & Braiker, 1981). Marlatt and Gordon (1985) and Sanchez-Craig and colleagues (Sanchez-Craig, Wilkinson, & Walker, 1987) reported that frustration in goal-directed activities (as well as the manner in which people deal with these frustrations) is the most common determinant of relapses. The choice between using a drug or not using it, moreover, has been shown to vary as a function of alternative enjoyable activities that are available to a person and barriers to these activities (Vuchinich & Tucker, 1988). In short, the ability to find emotional satisfaction nonchemically is a critical determinant of abstinence from substance abuse. Treatment that specifically helps patients develop enduring sources of emotional satisfaction as alternatives to substance use would appear to be highly promising. However, for many people with brain injury, the perceived value of using alcohol outweighs the negative consequences. Social situations become easier to handle, and lowered functional abilities can be attributed to intoxication (Langley, 1995).

This chapter presents information on the risks of developing substance abuse among people with neurologic dysfunction, and identification, prevention, and intervention strategies that can be implemented as part of rehabilitation and psychotherapy. Two treatment models shown to be effective with people with brain injury will be presented. The greatest opportunity for successful intervention comes when the clinician is able to artfully combine cognitive skill-based techniques with motivational approaches to provide the "how" and "why" for clients to change substance use patterns.

This chapter is organized around a public health prevention model that targets people at risk for a particular health problem, namely substance abuse, and intervenes at several levels. Typically in this prevention model, primary prevention refers to stopping a problem before it even begins. For most people with acquired brain injury, especially those who were under the influence of alcohol or other drugs at the time of injury, prevention begins at the level of secondary prevention, that is, the identification of the problem and implementation of strategies to limit its spread. Treatment is considered tertiary prevention; limiting the harm that is caused by an existing problem. The prevalence of substance abuse among people with acquired brain dysfunction demands the use of secondary and tertiary prevention strategies.

SECONDARY PREVENTION: SCREENING FOR RISK AND SYMPTOMS OF SUBSTANCE ABUSE

Screening Techniques: A Few Pointers

In general, use open-ended questions when asking about substance use. Ask questions that require more of an answer than a simple yes or no. Convey an open and nonjudgmental attitude; avoid confrontation and allow the person to save face when possible. Provide empathic responses that convey your goal of understanding so that you can best be of help to the person. Paraphrase a person's concerns to improve understanding and facilitate the exchange of information.

This information might be best obtained once you have established a working alliance or relationship with the client. Moreover, this information does not need to be garnered in one brief interview. Ask about the use of prescription medications as well as other drugs such as caffeine, nicotine, alcohol, and illicit drugs. Corroborate information with data from multiple sources, including background and collateral information, observations, physical examinations, and information from family and significant others. There is a high degree of concordance, typically greater than 90%, between self-report and family reports of substance use, yet in our clinical experiences, families often have a different perspective from clients on how use affects day-to-day functioning. To minimize resistance and defensiveness in the screening interview, it may be helpful to focus on historical questions and perspectives rather than query the person about current use and practices.

Screening for Risk Factors

The unique cognitive, emotional, behavioral, and physical impairments associated with brain injury create particular risks for alcohol and other drug use. Therapists and other rehabilitation professionals should be sensitive to these risks. Clientele and their families should be assessed for the presence of such risks. This can be done in interview format, or through the use of a thorough interdisciplinary evaluation that looks at all aspects of the person's functioning, including community and social climate. If preferred, a number of commercially available standardized questionnaires and assessment instruments are available for examining specific areas of risk, such as the Alcohol Expectancy Questionnaire (Brown, Christiansen, & Goldman, 1987) or the brief Michigan Alcohol Screening Test (Pokorney, Miller, & Kaplan, 1972). Following assessment, rehabilitation professionals should provide information and education to minimize risk and thus minimize AOD use.

Both pre- and postinjury risk factors need to be considered. Preinjury risk factors include premorbid AOD abuse, a life-style associated with the recreational use of AOD, limited knowledge of the potential dangers of substance use or an unwillingness to acknowledge these dangers, a family history or addiction or abuse, and a history of arrests or conviction of substance abuse related crimes, such as assault and battery, or driving while intoxicated.

Postinjury risks include both personal and environmental factors. Perhaps the most germane personal factor is the sense of social dislocation that occurs following acquired brain dysfunction and its rehabilitation. At its core, brain injury is profoundly isolating (Pollack, 1989). Weeks of acute care followed by extended rehabilitation result in a prolonged absence from the "real world" as one survivor of brain injury described it. "It was like I got caught out on an island, surrounded by rushing water. All my friends and family were in boats, sailing down the river away from me. I was stuck by myself. That's how lonely I felt," reported this 33-year-old man who was in coma for 3 months following a motorcycle crash. Loneliness and a desire to return to former social patterns can lead to increased risk of use, especially if the former life-style included activities that center around drinking or drug use (e.g., hanging out in a bar or tavern).

Reduced physical and cognitive abilities following acquired brain injury create unique stress and risk for substance use. One's ability to tolerate stress, frustration, and boredom is decreased following brain injury. There may be heightened sensitivity to stimulation and fatigue. Problem solving, memory, attention, and the ability to engage in constructive activity or interpersonal relationships may be impaired. These may all increase the risk of substance use. Diminished ability to accurately assess cause-and-effect relationships (which may occur in acquired brain injury) alone may contribute to the risk of making poor judgments about using alcohol or other drugs.

Many people with brain injury show limited social skills and limited coping skills. Some of these skill deficits may have existed preinjury, but cognitive and neurobehavioral sequelae of brain injury also may limit coping and social behavior. In general, people who are unable to engage in effective or adaptive problem solving or who have a limited repertoire of social skills are at risk for substance abuse. They may use alcohol or other drugs as a means of coping or relieving social anxiety. There are a number of coping instruments, including the Ways of Coping Questionnaire (Folkman & Lazarus, 1980) that can be used to formally assess coping skills.

Acquired brain injury often brings with it the burdens of loss and change. There may be a sudden reduction in abilities that may have been sources of pride and self-confidence. Elements of preinjury personality may be lost, leaving the person a stranger to self and loved ones. Brain injury can threaten or destroy vocational, romantic, athletic, artistic, social, familial and financial abilities.

Family stress may contribute to the increased substance use following brain injury. If the person with brain injury had been living with his or her family, separation during acute care and rehabilitation can be hard on family relationships. Communication can become difficult if the shared experience is disrupted. Role changes may occur. A person may go overnight from primary wage earner to dependent. The noninjured family members often need to assume additional family responsibilities, plus fit in time to visit and learn about the injured person's needs. Support once found within the family may become a scarce resource as the family system works to adapt to the changes.

Expectations and beliefs about the benefits of alcohol and other drug use may increase the chances that a person with brain injury will develop alcohol or other drug abuse. For example, if a person feels that alcohol can help her relax, then when she is stressed, she is more likely to use alcohol to excess. Some people believe that alcohol or other drugs help them "think clearer," feel "sexy," or "feel comfortable around people." These AOD expectancies motivate substance use and appear to be pervasive in our society. Research suggests that these beliefs may be deeply engrained. The stronger the expectation that alcohol or other drug use has positive benefits, the more at risk the person is for developing problems (Goldman, Brown, & Christiansen, 1987). The Alcohol Expectancy Questionnaire (Brown et al., 1987) can be used to formally assess a person's beliefs about alcohol use.

Social or environmental factors may also heighten a person's risk for developing substance problems. For example, societal misconceptions about people with disabilities in general (such as thinking that people with brain injury have pitiful lives and thus "deserve" to feel good in whatever way possible, including the use of alcohol or other drugs) add to the stress a person may feel following brain injury and may increase use. Conversely, the misconception that people with cognitive deficits have an inherent weakness, or can't be expected to cope well, may foster the notion that it is expected, in fact, seen as accepted, that people with brain injury can't handle stress and will turn to the quick fix. Lastly, many people believe that a person with brain dysfunction, particularly someone who was injured while intoxicated "must surely have learned his lesson" and "wouldn't do that again." For example, a neurologist who was working with a young, financially successful commodities trader did not want to refer this patient for substance abuse services, despite the fact that the patient had bilateral stroke in the frontal lobe secondary to cocaine use. The neurologist's reasoning was, "Surely he has learned his lesson and we don't want to stigmatize him—he's a young guy." The patient's reasoning for requesting treatment was, "I'll be sitting at home with nothing to do—except cocaine!" The nexus of these attitudes and misconceptions results in limited attention to the problem and consequently, limited accessibility to appropriate treatment, which in turn had the potential to intensify existing problems.

Closer to home, the tendency of family, friends, and even rehabilitation professionals, to ignore evidence of substance problems among people with brain dysfunction may stem from more than misinformation about these issues. Instead, this tendency may be "enabling" behavior. Enabling behaviors are words and actions that keep others from experiencing the full consequences of their alcohol and drug use, abuse, or dependence. Such enabling behaviors intensify the risk of substance abuse following brain injury. For example, one person with brain injury reported he did not see a problem with drinking beer at home—his mother bought it for him! When asked about the situation, mother reported that she indeed did buy beer for her son. This way, he was less likely to go out "looking for trouble," and "besides that, he tends to fall asleep early rather than complaining about how bored and depressed he is."

Screening for Symptoms

In addition to assessing a person's risk for developing alcohol problems, the therapist should evaluate the person's behavior for symptoms of substance abuse. The following symptom checklist was developed for the Resource Center for Substance Abuse Prevention and Disability by the Substance Abuse Resources and Disability (SARDI) Project (Moore, 1992) and includes substance abuse-related behaviors shown by people with disabilities. The presence of one or more of these symptoms is not necessarily indicative of substance abuse; however, if several of these symptoms are present, it suggests that issues related to alcohol and other drug use should be thoroughly explored and a full substance abuse assessment should be done.

Substance Abuse Checklist

- *Frequent intoxication:* Important information within this category includes the frequency of use or intoxication as well as the frequency of recreational activities which focus on drinking or drug use. For example, a client of day rehabilitation services for TBI reported that he "partied" four or five times per week. His family verified that he indeed hung out with the same group of friends he partied with prior to his injury. Although the client denied drinking to intoxication each time he met with his friends, he did admit to smoking dope on almost every occasion.

- *Use of atypical social settings:* Assessment of the settings in which substance use occurs includes asking about the person's immediate peer group, whether or not the person uses in isolation, and whether or not the person engages in social activities that do not include alcohol or other drugs. For example, the previously mentioned client did not have any other social contacts outside of "partying." If he was not hanging out, he was at home watching television alone in his room.
- *Intentional heavy use:* Inquiries under this category include information on whether the person drinks deliberately to get drunk, his or her tolerance level, and whether alcohol or other drug use is combined with prescription medications.
- *Symptomatic drinking:* Are there predictable patterns of use that are well known to others? Does the person rely on alcohol and other drugs to cope with stress? Does substance use remain constant across social contexts and during life-style changes?
- *Psychological dependence:* Information about the motivations for substance use can help identify psychological dependence on substance use. For example, one client reported that since her injury, she could not manage to attend school without taking extra codeine pain tablets to "not feel so jittery if the teacher calls on me and I can't remember the answer."
- *Health problems:* Does the person experience recurring physical conditions that may be associated with substance abuse? Did the person become disabled as a result of injury sustained under the influence of alcohol or other drugs? Does the person use substances despite taking anticonvulsant medication?
- *Job problems:* Often the presence of job-related problems can be indicative of ongoing substance abuse problems. Information about attendance, punctuality, and employment history can provide clues about substance abuse.
- *Problems with significant others:* Have important relationships been lost or damaged due to alcohol or other drug use? Have

family members or significant others expressed concern regarding the person's use?

- *Problems with the law or authority:* Although problems with the law or authorities around substance-related offenses (e.g., driving under the influence or disorderly conduct) can be direct indicators of substance use problems, other more subtle signs of substance abuse may be discerned in the person's attitude toward authority in general.
- *Financial problems:* Can the person account for spending money? Are payments made on time? Does the person frequently attempt to borrow money from peers, family, and staff?
- *Anger or belligerence:* Does the person act angry or defensive when asked about alcohol or other drug use?
- *Isolation:* Has the person become increasingly isolated from social contacts? Has there been a change in participation in social and family activities?
- *Handicappism:* Does the person blame all of his or her problems in life on the disability? Does the person focus on the disability to the exclusion of other personal aspects?

Brief Screening Tools

Two brief screening devices that are appropriate for use among people with neurologic dysfunction, and which can be easily incorporated during the information gathering process, are the RAFFT (Riggs & Alario, 1992) and the CAGE (Ewing, 1984), (see appendix A). Positive responses to any of these questions should be seen as a red flag, and further assessment of substance use patterns, beliefs, and expectations should be done.

TERTIARY PREVENTION: IDEAL INTERVENTION STRATEGIES FOR REDUCING SUBSTANCE ABUSE AMONG PEOPLE WITH BRAIN INJURY

As noted above, few specialized treatment programs for people with brain injury are available, and traditional treatment models are often insufficient to meet the needs of this population.

Cognitive and behavioral problems associated with brain dysfunction, such as memory problems, limited awareness, and communication difficulties, may interfere with traditional models of treatment delivery which often rely on verbal, insight oriented, group treatment modalities. For example, because of new learning difficulties, information may need to be presented several times and the timeframe for learning lengthened. The traditional 30-day program may be too short for learning and generalization to novel situations to take place, as individuals with brain dysfunction often fail to generalize learned behaviors to novel situations (Vogenthaler, 1987). Often, materials and methods may need to be concretized rather than being solely verbal or insight oriented. Methods that rely on self-awareness, including traditional psychotherapy and support group methods, may fail due to the person's inability to self-reflect or to perceive the effects of his or her behavior. Denial of deficits caused by brain dysfunction and those associated with substance abuse itself may be present but are often secondary to organic insightlessness rather than "denial" per se (Deaton, 1986; Fleming, Strong, & Ashton, 1996). "Denial" is a voluntary defense mechanism; people "choose" to ignore reality (Valliant, 1993). Substance abuse counselors who are unfamiliar with brain injury issues may not recognize the impact of cognitive issues on treatment participation and may see the person as noncompliant and unwilling to change.

The interplay between cognitive deficits and emotional denial may be seen in the following clinical vignette. A rehabilitation patient was admitted following frontal lobe injury sustained when the patient fell 30 feet at his workplace and fractured his skull. At the time of admission, his blood alcohol level was .15, well over the state's legal limit for intoxication. Throughout the course of the patient's inpatient rehabilitation stay, he denied "having trouble" or "having a problem" with alcohol, but was ready and willing to participate in an inpatient alcohol treatment because he felt he "needed help." However, he steadfastly denied "using" alcohol the day of his injury. The substance abuse counselor reported that he could not authorize treatment for the patient since the patient denied and refused to admit that he had a problem with alcohol. The patient's wife reported that she was reluctant to bring the patient home without substance abuse treatment because she felt that he might start up drinking again. She reported that the patient had been in substance abuse treatment about 12 years earlier, and occasionally "slipped" at home but it wasn't "much of a problem, not like he had before." Nevertheless, despite the staff's and family's concerns, the substance abuse counselor insisted that unless that patient admitted that he had a problem, treatment could not be authorized because "patients who deny they have problems do not succeed in our program." Rehabilitation staff intervened, and in a joint session with the substance abuse treatment provider and the patient, shifted the discussion from asking the patient to admit he had a problem to asking "if (he) had slipped" that day. The patient readily agreed that he had slipped but "wasn't using again, just had a few drinks with a friend for the holidays." The substance abuse counselor heard the patient's admission, and the patient began substance abuse treatment the next day. The patient's concrete reasoning and limited insight (secondary to frontal lobe injury), together with his self-belief that he was "not using," but only "having a few drinks, a slip," resulted in perceived "denial of alcohol problems." This case example stresses the importance not only of being aware of cognitive deficits that may interfere with intervention approaches, but also the need for collaboration between rehabilitation and substance abuse treatment professionals.

Ideal substance abuse interventions for people with brain dysfunction should be highly individualized. While experience working with people with brain injury is helpful, it is not always necessary. Jones (1992) noted that counselors who succeed with this population share two primary characteristics: creativity and client-centeredness. Creativity can be found in the therapist's willingness to be open to change in the means or route used to reach the client's stated goal, to let go of preconceptions, and to adapt conventional techniques to any particular client. Client-centeredness involves the capacity and willingness to meet the client at his or her level and to empower him or her to formulate goals to improve quality of life.

Other components and strategies which effective substance abuse interventions share with this population are: (1) Interdisciplinary services wherein a team of professionals with varied backgrounds and specialties work collaboratively to evaluate and treat the client's multiple, complex needs and facilitate growth in skills needed to achieve personal goals. (2) Concrete, goal-directed (versus psychodynamic) strategies. Many people with brain injury have limited insight or self-awareness. Effective strategies focus on the concrete here-and-now and focus on achievable goals that may lead to bigger goals. There is an emphasis on the development of specific skills relevant to the individual's day-to-day life. (3) Emphasis on the impact of substance use on functional–independent living skills. Most people with brain injury desire to live in the most independent manner possible and may benefit from education on how alcohol or other drug use interferes with independence. (4) Comprehensive and multidimensional programs address client needs on several levels including health, independent living skills, social and interpersonal skills, vocational needs, leisure and recreational skills, housing, financial needs, and family issues.

An exemplary program that offers specialized substance abuse intervention for people with disabilities, the Anixter Center in Chicago, has found that day-to-day concerns such as the need for reliable transportation or mentoring to attend community self-help groups create real obstacles to successful participation in treatment. To minimize external barriers, the Anixter Center uses case managers to coordinate auxiliary services such as transportation and eligibility for entitlements. Programing includes groups for improving social skills, academic skills, work adjustment skills, and communication in addition to individual and group substance abuse treatment. Participants have access to a health clinic that administers to the health needs of people with disabilities. Ongoing evaluation of this program suggested that the use of interdisciplinary services that support basic needs for daily living (e.g., health, housing, etc) allowed people with disabilities enough security and safety to actively engage in substance reduction protocols (Lorber, personal communication, May 24, 1996). The treatment program at the Anixter Center thus views substance abuse counseling as only one facet of the comprehensive program needed to help ameliorate substance abuse by people with brain dysfunction.

COLLABORATING WITH EXISTING TREATMENT PROGRAMS

In the absence of specific treatment programs for people with brain dysfunction, networking with existing community substance abuse programs is necessary. Collaboration and cross-agency cooperation is recommended to create resources to serve the unique needs of this group. Cross-training among agencies can increase the number of experts in the field. The brain injury rehabilitation professional can educate substance abuse professionals about the needs of people with brain injury. The substance abuse counselor can help the brain injury professional learn about prevention, intervention, and related issues.

This cross-training may be especially helpful in developing self-help and support groups for people with coexisting substance abuse and brain injury. These specialized groups may be necessary to adjust to the cognitive needs of people with cognitive dysfunction. Often, these people have difficulty with fatigue, complex attention, demands for rapid processing, and handling external distractions (Montgomery, 1995). According to the anecdotal reports of several clients who have brain injury, participation in nonadapted support group meetings can be frustrating, overwhelming, and shame-producing because they often feel as if they "can't keep up." For this reason, we try to link people to substance abuse support groups that are adapted to address cognitive dysfunction. In an effort to develop a larger number of socially accessible Alcoholics Anonymous groups in Chicago, we worked together with some of the volunteers who facilitate introductory Twelve Step groups at a major medical center. The introductory groups, entitled "How

It Works," provide an overview of Twelve Step meetings and
the principles of Alcoholics Anonymous. By providing information and consultation about brain injury and other disability
issues to the volunteers, we increased the opportunity that a
person with brain injury would be able to attend an introductory group that could be adapted to his or her needs. Qualita-
tive analysis of this collaboration showed that volunteer
substance abuse meeting leaders were receptive and welcomed
the opportunity to learn skills that would help them to be more
effective in individualizing programs.

Participation in self-help support groups for people in recovery can be very helpful. Most brain injury rehabilitation
programs have support groups for recovery from brain injury
issues. People in recovery for both brain injury and chemical
dependence generally should be linked to as many community
support services as available.

Corrigan, Lamb-Hart, and Rust (1995) described a pilot
program initiated in 1991 to increase collaboration among rehabilitation and substance abuse professionals to improve the
treatment efficacy for people who had experienced TBI. Called
the TBI Network, the model of treatment is community-based,
it uses an interdisciplinary staff with specialized knowledge of
brain injury to facilitate treatment by local substance abuse
professionals. Upon referral, clients are screened for their
likely eligibility (incurred a TBI with current sequelae and have
a history of substance abuse or are risk of same), and a small
amount of demographic information is recorded. Those who
are willing to participate and are appropriate for services receive a comprehensive assessment, which includes an independent interview of a family member when willing and available.
The primary method of subsequent intervention is resource
and service coordination to make linkages with existing substance abuse providers and sustain those linkages over the prolonged course of community integration. The TBI Network
uses case consultation to assist substance abuse program staff
to understand the unique strengths and weaknesses of an individual, adapt services and treatment plans to the individual's
abilities, trouble-shoot problems as they arise, and assist in

"wrapping around" other resources and services that individuals require to stabilize their health, financial, and vocational status. The large number of referrals to the program has indicated a marked need for the service, and initial evaluation data have shown positive behavior changes resulting from treatment. Because service provision is not facility-based, the program can be replicated with a minimum of start-up costs and can serve a large geographic region. Intervention of this type allows for maximal use of limited resources.

Within this type of collaboration, the TBI professional provides consultation to the substance abuse professional to adapt intervention to fit the specialized needs of the person with brain injury. The TBI professional can suggest different treatment modalities and can provide information about the individual's learning needs.

Two treatment protocols that have been field tested with people with brain injury will be described in the next section.

SPECIALIZED INTERVENTION PROTOCOLS FOR PEOPLE WITH BRAIN INJURY

Heinemann and colleagues (1995) field tested two models of substance abuse treatment (Skills Based Substance Abuse Prevention Counseling and Systematic Motivational Counseling), that had not been previously studied among people with brain injury, by applying interventions in a variety of treatment settings (e.g., outpatient rehabilitation, vocational training programs, residential services) to patients in different stages of recovery. Counseling techniques were designed to meet the unique needs of people with brain injury, including accommodations for cognitive impairments, motivational difficulties, and behavioral impairments. Often, such persons are not admitted to traditional treatment programs. The substance abuse interventions were incorporated into persons' existing brain injury rehabilitation programs, and various members of the team were instrumental in its delivery. Information about each intervention follows.

SKILLS BASED SUBSTANCE ABUSE PREVENTION COUNSELING

Mervin Langley described Skills Based Substance Abuse Prevention Counseling (SBSAPC) in 1991 and 1995 publications on prevention of alcohol-related problems after traumatic brain injury. Dr. Langley's method involves four stages of treatment: comprehensive evaluation, motivational enhancement, coping skill training, and structured generalization. All techniques utilized in this approach are based on strategies already found effective among non-brain-injured persons. The basic premise of the model is that the risk of abusing substances as a coping mechanism is heightened for people with brain injury, and techniques target areas that contribute to this problem.

As reviewed above, several neuropsychological deficits, such as impaired learning and generalization, and impaired insight and awareness, may lessen the utility of conventional treatment approaches. Langley's SBSAPC is expressly directed toward circumventing these aspects of neuropsychological impairment. Clients learn by rehearsing cognitive and coping skills rather than obtaining information through traditional education. Awareness deficits are addressed by systematically increasing problem recognition, by retraining self-monitoring abilities, and by selecting techniques that do not rely on awareness for their success. Impulse control deficits are dealt with by extinguishing or counterconditioning reactivity to substance cues and by increasing self-control under protected stimulus conditions.

Interventions progress through four overlapping stages. In the first stage, comprehensive evaluation, measures are completed which guide the selection of treatment targets and provide baseline data for determining the effectiveness of the strategies. Homework is introduced which facilitates self-monitoring abilities. In stage 2, motivational enhancement, the focus is on strengthening decision-making abilities. Stage 3, coping skill training, provides training in neurocognitive and coping skills for making changes happen. Finally, in stage 4, or generalization, newly learned behaviors are transferred to real-world settings. Each component has highly structured techniques that occur within a collaborative client–therapist relationship.

Within the collaboration of client and therapist, personal feedback about the interaction of substance use and neurocognitive and motor impairments offers the best hope for behavior change. The challenge for the clinician is to provide information that relates to deficits the client acknowledges as legitimate. For example, a person with balance problems may be given information about the effects of alcohol on cerebellar function for coordinated movement. The goal in this process of "motivational interviewing" is to establish dissonance between the person's substance use behavior and important personal goals (Miller, 1985). The clinician must thoroughly understand the client's actual and perceived deficits as well as goals. Identifying and formulating achievable short- and long-term goals is a prerequisite to success and provides a rationale for modifying substance use.

Techniques used in SBSAPC include establishing a working relationship, providing highly personalized feedback that creates a discrepancy between important goals and substance use behaviors, and managing positive outcome expectancies. In addition, SBSAPC techniques help clients recognize that beliefs mediate substance use, develop counters to positive substance use beliefs, practice countering skills, identify personal high-risk situations, determine strengths and weaknesses in high-risk situations, and practice coping responses in high-risk situations. Teaching clients to cope with cue exposures requires caution. There is a fine line between allowing a client to rehearse skills in cue situations and allowing the client to indulge in substance use fantasies. Several procedural safeguards are suggested, including revising the abstinence contract, ending cue sessions with successful use of skills which facilitates a reduction in subjective desire to use, and using cues which the client is likely to experience within the course of a normal week. Powerful cues, such as the direct use of substances, should be avoided in favor of symbolic presentations such as pictures or imagery.

Evaluation of the effectiveness of this program showed that participants whose alcohol coping skills increased from baseline to reassessment were more likely to have become abstinent over time than those who did not show a change. Analysis of the treatment components showed that preparatory interventions, such as conceptualization, goal-setting, discussion of costs and benefits of substance use, instructions, modeling, and feedback were represented to a greater extent than skill rehearsal. The benefits obtained from coping skill training were the result of personally relevant information, instruction, and demonstration rather than the clients' actual performance of the skills during sessions. By making information about substance use effects relevant to the person in his or her personal life situation, treatment appeared more effective than when information is provided generally. Cognitive deficits that are associated with the failure of traditional information giving, such as abstraction, attention, and memory deficits are circumvented by the addition of interventions that link information with day-to-day functional skills.

Systematic Motivational Counseling

Several current theories of substance abuse (Cox & Klinger, 1988; Marlatt, 1985; Miller, 1985), hinge on the concept of "motivation." Motivation refers to the balance between the satisfaction that a person expects to obtain by using substances and the emotional satisfaction that he or she expects to find from nonchemical sources. A motivational intervention is one that shifts this balance by increasing the person's "probability of entering, continuing, and complying with an active change strategy" (Miller, 1985, p. 88). Systematic Motivational Counseling (SMC) specifically targets persons' motivation for recovery. Miranti, Cox, Klinger, and colleagues adapted this technique for use with people with brain injury as part of the federally funded field test coordinated by Heinemann et al.

(1995). They found that SMC techniques can be used success-fully with people with brain injury by focusing jointly on indi-viduals' motivation for recovery from brain injury and substance abuse alike.

Systematic motivational counseling is based on Cox and Klinger's (1988) motivational model of substance use. Defini-tions of basic motivational principles will facilitate understand-ing of this model. First, *affect* is the experiential or psychological component of an emotional response. Motivational theorists think of affect being either positive or negative. Positive affect means pleasurable engagement with the environment whereas negative affect is unpleasurable. *Affective change* is a change in affect from its present state, and most people are motivated to change negative affect to positive affect. Substances often are used to achieve affective change. An *incentive* is any object or event that a person expects will bring about an affective change. Incentives can be positive (things the person wants to obtain) or negative (things the person wishes to avoid). Every goal is an incentive, but not every incentive is a goal. For example, a woman with brain injury might expect that having a million dollars would increase her positive affect, but will not be com-mitted to having a million dollars because that may be un-achievable. A *current concern* is a person's motivational state between the time a decision is made to pursue an incentive and the time the goal is reached or relinquished. During this time, people appear vigilant to cues that have an impact on obtaining their goals. Many current concerns may be operative at the same time.

This motivational model illuminates the principles by which substances or other nonchemical events can be incen-tives for people. Motivations to pursue nonchemical incentives to bring about affective change may also govern substance use. The relative balance between chemical and nonchemical incen-tives is a critical determinant of the motivation to use alcohol. Systematic motivational counseling operates on the idea that it is possible to empower people to increase their nonchemical sources of emotional satisfaction that are incompatible with substance use, thereby shifting the balance in favor of decisions not to use.

Getting Started

The therapist who intends to use SMC will spend some time initially becoming acquainted with the client, establishing rapport, and beginning to establish a therapeutic bond. For clients with brain injuries, this process may be lower than with persons without cognitive impairments. The therapist also introduces SMC by explaining its rationale and eliciting the client's reactions to determine if he or she wants to proceed. Assuming that there is a desire to go forward, the therapist then begins to understand the client's motivations for substance use and how this relates to other areas in life. Some areas to be explored include the circumstances surrounding the beginning of counseling, the person's history of substance use, the client's view of the problem and his or her goals for counseling.

Systematic motivational counseling is initiated by assessing people's motivational patterns through the use of the Motivational Structure Questionnaire (Cox, Klinger, & Blount, 1996). The technique is an individualized one that does not use a session-by-session agenda that is identical for all clients. Although certain components are used with all clients, others may or may not be used with specific clients, depending on their motivational characteristics.

Preliminary counseling components include reviewing the individual's MSQ to review goals and analyzing the interrelationships among goals. Goal-setting is the next component, and treatment goals are established. Goal ladders, with short-term, session-to-session goals determined to achieve major long-term goals, are constructed. Subsequent sessions focus on improving the client's ability to meet goals and resolving the conflicts among goals. There is also focus on empowering clients to disengage from inappropriate goals and identifying new incentives.

In SMC, the therapist also works with the client to move to achieve more positive goals than to avoid negative goals, as this kind of appetitive life-style is seen as psychologically satisfying. For some clients, this may be accomplished by cognitive reframing to help them focus on positive aspects of their goals rather than negative aspects. In other cases, more success might be gained by helping clients reduce the number of negative concerns in their lives. Associated with this is an effort to help people reexamine their sources of self-esteem. Low self-esteem is a pervasive problem for people with substance abuse as well as people with brain injury. Some people tend to hold high standards for themselves and are unduly harsh on themselves when they are unable to achieve them (Klinger, 1977). This may be especially true for people with brain injury who cling to the image of themselves before the injury, and who because of neurocognitive and motor impairments, are no longer able to perform activities that they once did with ease. This self-condemnation, of not being satisfied with current achievements because they do not seem commensurate with previous achievements, is often seen among people with brain injury who continue to abuse substances and presents a major barrier to adjustment. Thus, counselors try to assist clients find new ways of feeling good about themselves, to become less self-condemning and to develop self-forgiveness for goals they have not attained.

Field evaluation of this model with people with brain injury showed that approximately 20% of people became abstinent and 41% maintained abstinence during treatment. Participants showed significantly fewer concerns and greater movement toward an appetitive life-style than did the no-treatment control group.

CONCLUSIONS

People with brain injury are at particular risk for resuming or starting substance abuse. Providing skills and counseling to reduce risks is but one approach. Such abuse may be maintained as a coping mechanism or means of achieving positive affect. Successful substance abuse treatment for people with brain injury requires accommodation of neurocognitive and other neuropsychological impairments, but can be achieved, especially when treatment is part of a multidisciplinary approach to brain injury rehabilitation. Two models of treatment, a skills based substance abuse prevention model, and a model of motivational counseling, have been field tested and shown to be useful in this population. An ideal treatment modality would target both skill deficits and motivational concerns.

Therapists who work with people with brain injury recognize the need for specialized services. However, because few specialized services are available, brain injury rehabilitation professionals will find it prudent to learn as much as possible about the subject. Such knowledge enables the professional to consult effectively with substance abuse professionals to customize available interventions to meet the needs of any particular client. A collaboration between brain injury and substance abuse professionals was described as one means of delivering services to people with brain injury. Skillful blending of cognitive and motivational treatments and judicious application of substance abuse interventions, offer great promise in helping people with brain injury adjust and improve their quality of life.

REFERENCES

American Psychiatric Association (1994). *Diagnostic and statistical manual of mental disorders* (4th ed.). Washington, DC: Author.

Boyle, M. J., Vella, L., & Moloney, E. (1991). Role of drugs and alcohol in patients with head injury. *Journal of the Royal Society of Medicine, 84,* 608–610.

Brown, S. A., Christiansen, B. A., & Goldman, M. S. (1987). The Alcohol Expectancy Questionnaire: An instrument for the assessment of adolescent and adult alcohol expectancies. *Journal of Studies of Alcohol, 48,* 483–491.

Collins, J. F. (1990). *Types of injuries by selected characteristics: United States 1985–87.* National Center for Health Statistics, Vital Health Statistics, 10, 185.

Corrigan, J. D., Lamb-Hart, G. L., & Rust, E. (1995). A programme of intervention for substance abuse following traumatic brain injury. *Brain Injury, 9,* 221–236.

Corrigan, J. D., Rust, E., & Lamb-Hart, G. L. (1995). The nature and extent of substance abuse problems in persons with traumatic brain injury. *Journal of Head Trauma Rehabilitation, 10,* 29–46.

Cox, W. M., & Klinger, E. (1988). A motivational model of alcohol use. *Journal of Abnormal Psychology, 97,* 168–180.

Cox, W. M., Klinger, E., & Blount, J. (1996). Structured Motivational Questionnaire. In *NIAAA Addiction measurement tools.* Washington, DC: National Institute of Alcoholism and Alcohol Abuse.

Deaton, A. V. (1986). Denial in the aftermath of traumatic brain injury: Its manifestations, measurement and treatment. *Rehabilitation Psychology, 31,* 231–240.

Donovan, D. M., & Chaney, E. F. (1985). Alcoholic relapse prevention and intervention: Models and methods. In G. A. Marlatt & J. R. Gordon (Eds.), *Relapse prevention: Maintenance strategies in the treatment of addictive behaviors.* New York: Guilford.

Dunlop, T. W., Udvarhelyi, G. B., Stedem, A. F., & O'Connor, J. M. (1991). Comparison of patients with and without emotional/ behavioral deterioration during the first year after traumatic brain injury. *Journal of Neuropsychiatry and Clinical Neurosciences, 3,* 150–156.

Ewing, J. A. (1984). Detecting alcoholism: The CAGE questionnaire. *Journal of the American Medical Association, 252,* 27–29.

Fleming, J. M., Strong, J., & Ashton, R. (1996). Self-awareness of deficits in adults with traumatic brain injury: How to best measure? *Brain Injury, 10,* 1–15.

Folkman, S., & Lazarus, R. S. (1980). An analysis of coping in a middle-aged community sample. *Journal of Health and Social Behavior, 21,* 219–239.

Goldman, M. S., Brown, S. A., & Christiansen, B. A. (1987). Expectancy theory: Thinking about drinking. In H. T. Bland & K. E. Leonard (Eds.), *Psychological theories of drinking and alcoholism* (pp. 181–226). New York: Guilford.

Heinemann, A. W., Cox, M., Blount, J., Klinger, E., Miranti, S. V., Ridgely, M., Langley, M., & Schmidt, M. F. (1995). *Final report: Substance abuse as a barrier to employment following traumatic brain injury.* Chicago, IL: Rehabilitation Institute of Chicago.

Jones, G. A. (1992). Substance abuse treatment for persons with brain injuries: Identifying models and modalities. *NeuroRehabilitation, 2,* 27–34.

Kiley, D. J., Heinemann, A. W., Doll, M., Shade-Zeldow, Y., Roth, E., & Yarkony, G. (1992). Rehabilitation professionals' knowledge and attitudes about substance abuse. *NeuroRehabilitation, 2,* 35–44.

Klinger, E. (1977) *Meaning and void: Inner experience and the incentives in people's lives.* Minneapolis: University of Minnesota Press.

Kreutzer, J. S., Doherty, K. R., Harris, J. A., & Zasler, N. D. (1990). Alcohol use among persons with traumatic brain injury. *Journal of Head Trauma Rehabilitation, 5,* 9–20.

Kreutzer, J. S., Wehman, P. H., Harris, J. A., Burns, C. T., & Young, H. F. (1991). Substance use and crime patterns among persons with traumatic brain injury referred for supported employment. *Brain Injury, 5,* 177–187.

Kreutzer, J. S., Witol, A. D., & Marwitz, J. H. (1996). Alcohol and drug use among young persons with traumatic brain injury. *Journal of Learning Disabilities, 29,* 643–651.

Langley, M. J. (1991). Preventing post-injury alcohol-related problems: A behavioral approach. In B. T. McMahon & L. R. Shaw (Eds.), *Work worth doing: Advances in brain injury rehabilitation* (pp. 251–275). Orlando, FL: Paul M. Deutsch Press.

Langley, M. J. (1995). *Preventing alcohol-related problems after traumatic brain injury: A behavioral approach.* Chicago: Rehabilitation Institute of Chicago.

Langley, M. J., & Kiley, D. (1992). Prevention of substance abuse in persons with neurological disabilities. *NeuroRehabilitation, 2,* 56–64.

Marlatt, G. A. (1985). Cognitive assessment and intervention procedures for relapse prevention. In G. A. Marlatt & J. R. Gordon (Eds.), *Relapse prevention: Maintenance strategies in the treatment of addictive behaviors.* New York: Guilford.

Marlatt, G. A., & Gordon, J. R. (1985). *Relapse prevention: Maintenance strategies in the treatment of addictive behaviors.* New York: Guilford.

McLellan, B. A., Vingilis, E., Larkin, E., Stoduto, G., Filgate, M., & Sharkey, P. W. (1993). Psychosocial characteristics and follow-up of drinking and non-drinking drivers in motor vehicle crashes. *Journal of Trauma, 35,* 245–250.

Miller, W. R. (1985). Motivation for treatment: A review with special emphasis on alcoholism. *Psychological Bulletin, 98,* 84–107.

Montgomery, G. K. (1995). A multi-factor account of disability after brain injury: Implications for neuropsychological counseling. *Brain Injury, 9,* 453–469.

Moore, D. (1992). Substance abuse assessment and diagnosis in medical rehabilitation. *NeuroRehabilitation, 2,* 7–15.

Murray, P. K. (1987). Clinical pharmacology in rehabilitation. In B. Caplan (Ed.), *Rehabilitation psychology desk reference* (pp. 501–525). Rockville, MD: Aspen.

National Foundation for Brain Research (1994). *Annual Summary.* Washington, DC: Author.

Parsons, O. A. (1987). Intellectual impairment in alcoholics. *Acta Medica Scandinavica, 717,* 33–46.

Pokorney, A. D., Miller, B. A., & Kaplan, H. B. (1972). The MAST. A shortened version of the Michigan Alcoholism Screening Test. *American Journal of Psychiatry, 129,* 342–345.

Polich, J. M., Armor, D. J., & Braiker, H. B. (1981). *The course of alcoholism: Four years after treatment.* New York: Wiley.

Pollack, I. W. (1989). Traumatic brain injury and the rehabilitation process: A psychiatric perspective. In D. W. Ellis & A. L. Christensen (Eds.), *Neuropsychological treatment after brain injury* (pp. 56–81). Norwell, MA: Kluwer Academic.

Riggs, A., & Alario, M. (1992). *RAFFT.* Washington, DC: VSA Educational, Resource Center for Substance Abuse and Disability.

Sanchez-Craig, M., Wilkinson, D. A., & Walker, K. (1987). Theory and methods for secondary prevention of alcohol problems: A cognitive approach. In W. M. Cox (Ed.), *Treatment and prevention of alcohol problems. A resource manual* (pp. 100–132). Orlando, FL: Academic Press.

Schmidt, M. F., & Garvin, L. J. (1994). Substance abuse patterns one year after inpatient rehabilitation. Poster presented at the National Head Injury Eleventh Annual Meeting, Chicago, Illinois.

Sparadeo, F. R., Strauss, D., & Barth, J. T. (1990). The incidence, impact and treatment of substance abuse in head trauma rehabilitation. *Journal of Head Trauma Rehabilitation, 5,* 1–8.

Tucker, J. A., Vuchinich, R. E., & Harris, C. V. (1985). Determinants of substance abuse relapse. In M. Galizio & S. A. Maisto (Eds.), *Determinants of substance abuse: Biological, psychological, and environmental factors* (pp. 158–214). New York: Plenum.

Vailliant, G. E. (1983). *The natural course of alcoholism. Causes, patterns and paths to recovery.* Cambridge, MA: Harvard University Press.

Vailliant, G. E. (1993). *The wisdom of the ego.* Cambridge, MA: Harvard University Press.

Vogenthaler, D. R. (1987). An overview of head injury: Its consequences and rehabilitation. *Brain Injury, 1,* 113–127.

Vuchinich, R. E., & Tucker, J. A. (1988). Contributions from behavioral theories of choice to an analysis of alcohol abuse. *Journal of Abnormal Psychology, 97,* 181–195.

APPENDIX A: SCREENING INSTRUMENTS

The **RAFFT** (Riggs & Alano, 1992) includes these questions:

- Have you ever drank or used drugs to **R**elax, feel better about yourself, or fit in?
- Have you ever drank or used drugs while you were by yourself, **A**lone?
- Do any of your closest **F**riends drink or use drugs?
- Does a close **F**amily member have a problem with alcohol or drug use?
- Have you ever gotten into **T**rouble from drinking or drug use?

The **CAGE** (Ewing, 1988) is named for the first letters of the boldface words in the following questions:

- Have you ever decided to **C**ut down your drinking (or drug use)?
- Have you ever felt **A**nnoyed because of criticism of your drinking (or use)?
- Have you ever felt **G**uilty about your use of alcohol (or other drugs)?
- Have you ever had an **E**ye-opener in the morning (morning drinking or use)?

Name Index

Subject Index

245